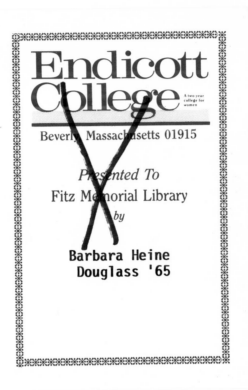

Social Survival
for Children

A TRAINER'S RESOURCE BOOK

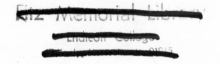

Social Survival for Children

A TRAINER'S RESOURCE BOOK

By

Peter W. Dowrick, Ph.D.

BRUNNER/MAZEL, *Publishers* • New York

Library of Congress Cataloging-in-Publication Data

Dowrick, Peter W.
  Social Survival for children.

  Bibliography: p. 247
  Includes indexes.
  1. Social skills in children. 2. Social interaction
in children. 3. Social skills in children – Therapeutic
use. 4. Child psychotherapy. I. Title.
[DNLM: 1. Interpersonal Relations. 2. Social
Behavior Disorders – in infancy & childhood. 3. Social
Behavior Disorders – therapy. WS 350.8.S6 D751s]
BF723.S62D68 1986   155.4'18   86-11797
ISBN 0-87630-432-3

Copyright © 1986 by Peter W. Dowrick

Published by
BRUNNER/MAZEL, INC.
19 Union Square West
New York, New York 10003

MANUFACTURED IN THE UNITED STATES OF AMERICA

To Jamie
whose social survival as a young child
made it seem so easy and so much fun.

Contents

vii

Preface

RATIONALE

The purpose of this book is simple. It is to provide descriptions of a variety of social skills training procedures accessible to clinicians and other providers of child care. It is also to present the procedures in a context of "social skills" interpreted more comprehensively than before. Social functioning is crucial for childhood well-being in ways that go beyond repercussions of the important but narrowly conceived poles of shyness and aggression. So it seems timely to begin to draw together knowledge and procedures of more diverse conditions – including populations with special needs, such as those created by sensory deficits, and with disorders secondarily influenced by social dysfunction, such as illness or psychopathology.

My philosophy throughout is that social skills training (indeed any therapeutic intervention) should provide a child with more choice. That is, children can be trained in skills and the confidence to use those skills, for what they *can* do, not what they *ought* to do, in a variety of stressful situations. Suitably guided, the child may then discover options which allow a more mutually rewarding interaction with the world.

Five years ago there were almost no books available that described procedures for social skills training with children. This book was originally conceived to fill that void. If written immediately it might well have treated the subject matter of social skills and assertiveness quite similarly to that already documented in books for adult populations. However, a variety of tasks allowed me to compile my ideas but slowly and delayed my settling into the manuscript. In the meantime a trickle of books – some of them praiseworthy – have appeared to review and describe the training of social skills in children; a number of others have included chapters on childhood aggression or social withdrawal (see Bibliography at the end of this book). These publications reflect the considerable growth in attention to the field.

To many readers social skills training will be equated with programs to ameliorate childhood aggression or social withdrawal as the identified problems. These issues will remain critical to the area, and there will always be a need for books that contain better descriptions of these conditions and the associated treatments. But it now seems most timely in 1986 to consider a more comprehensive interrelationship between social functioning and childhood well-being. Through this book I offer a somewhat concise attempt to broaden the concept of social skills training, around a focus of the contribution of social interaction in the maintenance or dissipation of a variety of conditions. The emphasis is more on solutions than on causes.

OVERVIEW

The content of the book is, primarily, concerned with the pragmatics of intervention. Thus the first two chapters, while reviewing the manifestations of effective social interactions and the consequences of ineffective functioning, emphasize the different techniques available for achieving change. There are implications for the selection of a variety or a combination of approaches, details of which are illustrated in subsequent chapters.

The following three chapters cover the most traditional domain of social skills intervention – withdrawal and aggression – with one difference. A distinction is drawn between the social anxiety of shyness and social "phobias," the specificity of the latter demanding a very different approach to treatment. In each of these and subsequent chapters (through Chapter 10) one or more intervention strategy is described in reasonable detail and illustrated with selected case studies or program descriptions. A match between strategies and chapters was made to reduce repetition throughout the book. The matchings were determined on the basis of logical and frequent use of interventions within specific circumstances (e.g., filmed models for socially withdrawn children, conflict resolution for dysfunctional families). However, it is to be emphasized that all interventions, some in particular, have multiple applicability. Most problems are more effectively treated through a combined, comprehensive intervention approach.

Chapters 6–10 deal with further specific circumstances, critical to the social functioning of children. Chapter 6 describes primarily family issues, in which I take the view that the training of parents in "child management" essentially serves to develop social skills in the parent — that is, more consistent, coherent communication with the child. In Chapter 7, the role of assertiveness and other social skills is examined in the context of children who may need to escape sexual or physical harassment — a topic specialized and sensitive enough to warrant a short chapter of its own. Chapters 8 and 9 cover a gamut of special populations — for example, children with medical or psychological disorders, those with physically or mentally handicapping conditions. The interrelationship between these conditions and social functioning deserves attention beyond that which it has already received: it may well provide the fastest emerging speciality area in the field over the next 5 years.

All issues and procedures in the book have their own or modified applicability to all ages of children. However, a modest correlation exists between a child's age and the likelihood of some problems to be recognized and attended to. There is a slight tendency for the order of topics in Chapters 3–6 to reflect this chronology. By adolescence certain developmental and social circumstances bring forth issues of relevance, to which Chapter 10 is devoted. In particular, programs are described for the prevention and rehabilitation of delinquency, in which social interaction is a single but frequently critical factor of importance.

The most important technological accessory to social skills training is the subject of Chapter 11. My own work over the last 10 years with social skills, children, and other concerns and populations has convinced me of the value of video in this context. This attitude is not only my own bias, however, as the routine mention of video recording has noticeably increased in reports describing social skills training in the last 2 or 3 years. The more ready availability of equipment (and its less daunting technicality, ironically) has further increased the need to understand the methods and the implications of using this instrument. The final chapter offers philosophical and practical guidelines for interventions broadly considered. Issues raised include concern for efficacy and ethics, as well as the delineation of responsibilities and frameworks of change.

ACKNOWLEDGMENTS

If I had to pick out two people from the many who have influenced me in this book, I would choose Albert Bandura and Todd Risley. Dr. Bandura provided me with some fundamental thinking in my early work with children; Dr. Risley, through his clinical innovations and most recently as a colleague, has frequently prompted better interpretations of what I have tried to understand. I appreciate them both, different as they are, for their science and their sense. I also note my special appreciation for colleagues in Auckland where the background to this work began, and colleagues in London and Anchorage who encouraged me to continue. And I extend warm gratitude to many students and research assistants (several whose names are cited within) who helped me review, revise, and implement many of the ideas in this book.

Peter W. Dowrick
Anchorage, Alaska

Social Survival
for Children

A TRAINER'S RESOURCE BOOK

CHAPTER 1

What Are Social Skills in Children?

A remarkable feature of the social skills training field is its recency. Given our current familiarity with the term *social skills* and its close relative *assertiveness*, it is surprising to think that 20 years ago these terms were rare. In his book, *Psychology and Social Problems* (1964), Michael Argyle, a social psychologist at Oxford University, devoted but one paragraph to social skills. There he remarked on the growth of the area, concluding: "It is possible that methods could be devised for training . . . " (p. 34). It is true that methods of training social skills were already developing in other parts of the world, but it is more important to note that he subsequently became, in a very short time, a leader in the field. A major contribution is his research on eye contact – or what he prefers to call mutual gaze. Another leader in the field was Argyle's associate at Oxford, Peter Trower; in the United States, Robert Liberman from Los Angeles made particular contributions to social skills training for people with schizophrenic disorders, while Alan Bellack and others in Pittsburgh spawned numerous research studies examining the problems of generalization and maintenance in assertiveness training.

Assertiveness as a popular movement probably began in 1970 with the first edition of the Alberti and Emmons book, *Your Perfect Right*. Later a specialty submovement of women's assertiveness began, very much influenced by the work of Patricia Jakubowski. Most recently, practitioners and researchers turned their attention to social interaction skills of children. Notable contributors to the field include Cartledge and Milburn for their work in the educational setting, Goldstein and associates for an approach called *structured learning*, Shure and Spivack for a problem-solving training approach to social interaction, Bash and Camp for their "think aloud" program, and Hops and his associates for their work with withdrawn and isolate children. In the last few years, attention to the field has increased, including some diversification into more specialized populations (e.g., emotionally disturbed and developmentally disabled). Some major contributors do not refer to "social skills," though their work clearly focuses on issues of social functioning. In short, it has become increasingly difficult to identify a short list of "leaders" in social skills training with children.

A consequence of the recent and rapid development of the field is that the enthusiasm for practice has often outstripped the theoretical or research underpinnings. However, development in the field has now reached a point where these deficits are more systematically becoming rectified. (Works of selected authors will be reviewed where appropriate throughout the book.)

The value for children in being socially skilled cannot be underestimated. Not only are there benefits, many of which are obvious, for the socially adept, but there are penalties and repercussions for the socially inept. The repercussions are not as obvious and much research is currently aimed at the sometimes subtle and obscure links between the socially awkward child and the psychologically disturbed adult. Whether we approve or not, humans are social beings. Social interactions are almost ubiquitous aspects of our lives – play, learning, and work – and often sought out, not just treated as inevitable. Children who are socially skilled have more fun. They get more enjoyment from what they are engaged in, and they exercise more choice over what they do. Unskilled children may be victimized by their peers in various ways and neglected or abused by adults.

In this chapter, attention is given first to an attempt to describe the nature of children's social skills: discussion of definitions and description of components. This section will be followed by an outline of the normal development of social skills and the major consequences of poor development of these skills. By implication, the preventive possibilities of training seem to be far-reaching and obvious. Research bearing on these issues will be briefly examined, including an analysis of specific skill components (see p. 11).

DEFINITIONS OF TERMS

Numerous and various definitions exist for the term *social skills*. Some of the most frequently cited will be listed here, leading to a brief analysis of the essentials to be included or at least implied in any operational definition.

Perhaps the most often quoted definition is that by Combs and Slaby (1977): "the ability to interact with others in a given social context in specific ways that are socially acceptable or valued and at the same time personally beneficial, mutually beneficial, or beneficial primarily to others" (p. 162). This definition points out that not only is the context social and the behavior skillful, but the social transaction is aimed at personal benefits for the parties concerned. A definition of Libet and Lewinsohn (1973) describes the social skill as "the complex ability both to emit behaviors that are positively or negatively reinforced and not to emit behaviors that are punished or extinguished by others" (p. 304), a contrast more in terminology than in content. Phillips's (1978) more voluminous definition states: "the extent to which he or she can communicate with others, in a manner that fulfills one's rights, requirements, satisfactions, or obligations to a reasonable degree without damaging the other persons' similar rights, requirements, satisfactions, or obligations, and hopefully shares these rights, etc. with others in free and open exchange." More succinctly Lange and Jakubowski (1976) refer to " . . . expressing thoughts, feelings, and beliefs in direct, honest, and appropriate ways which do not violate another person's rights." This definition was intended more to describe assertiveness than social skills, yet it seems to say no less than that of Phillips.

All these definitions seem to err towards being too broad. That is, for the most part they appear to include all, or at least most, of the events that are considered social skills, but also to include many things that are not social skills. For example, Combs and Slaby's definition seems not to exclude nonsocial elements of interactive games. Whereas chess and baseball do involve social skills, these skills are generally considered to be distinct from the ability to follow King's Gambit or to hit home runs. And, to be perfectly bizarre, could not the argument be made that the act of suicide, as an expression of anguish, might be contrived to fit Lange and Jakubowski's description of assertiveness? The argument would be defeated, I hope, but the definition remains overly inclusive. (Although it may startle the logic in most modern cultures, suicide may be seen as quite genuinely assertive, in, say traditional Japan – reminding us of important cultural differences.)

However, for psychologists or trainers, whose primary concern is to work with children rather than with abstractions, an overinclusive definition is a useful and appropriate place to start. It provides content information that enables people to generate many examples spontaneously. To avoid disagreements, we then build onto our general definition to make it suitably specific; we create an *operational definition* to suit our particular circumstances. That is, for the identified children we are working with, we can specify the types of actions and reactions that are adaptive and appropriate to their context. The operational definition, then, applies to limited settings, but is consonant with a general definition. The challenge of complete generality with exhaustive and exclusive properties is left to the philosophers.

An operational definition should embrace the following three properties: social skills are interpersonal, purposeful, and learnable (cf. discussion by Hargie, Saunders, & Dickson, 1981).

Social skills are interpersonal and interrelated. The types of social settings that are to be addressed must first be clarified: Who might be involved in the interchange, what relationships exist between them, what is the larger context? Second, social skillfulness does not occur in a vacuum, but an individual has control over only his or her part of the action. Therefore, judgement and flexibility are necessary. When we communicate we must ask, what do we want the other party to know, what do they want to know, what do they want us to know?

Social skills are purposeful and self-controlled. The benefits of the interaction must be understood. Is it an issue of persuasion, is it more blessed to send than to receive, will facts or feelings give satisfaction? Furthermore, there is a goal of individual choice. Assertiveness, for example, should be exercised as an option, not as an obligation; a child who wishes to remain in a corner absorbed in a book, should feel free to do so – but out of choice, not through lack of ability to join the other children playing outside (cf. the title *The Assertive Option* of the book by Jakubowski and Lange, 1978).

Social skills comprise units of learnable behavior. The barrier to skillful and enjoyable exchange may not be the inability to recognize the eventual solution as often as the confusing complexity of where to begin. Therefore, a task analysis that breaks down a macroskill into manageable components is essential. Making conversation with a stranger (macroskill) includes the approach, body language, eye contact, voice control, identifying what to say, asking open-ended questions, and handing conversation back and forth – among other things. Some of the components will be in the repertoire, others can be trained individually, and then all can be assembled and integrated.

COMPONENTS

The various aspects of social interaction are so diverse and complex that it pays to consider them along different dimensions: Three useful themes are the *attributes* of the skill, the *situations* that they serve, and the personal *processes* involved. Any social episode will occur as an intersection of these dimensions, but training may be organized differentially along the dimensions.

Attributes

The most basic attribute of social skill is *openness*. When communication is open, it implies not only being forthright but being receptive to the other person. It implies honesty and encourages trust. As a personality trait, openness is valued in most societies, particularly in the United States.

Another attribute that facilitates social exchange is *friendliness*. This conveys more emotional properties than openness. Further, it demands a level of receptivity to other people's emotions, enabling judgement of when paradoxical friendliness – for example, teasing or being coy – is appropriate.

Assertiveness is a attribute that goes beyond facilitating openness and flirts with control. With its emphasis on expressiveness, it also goes beyond the warm emotions of friendliness to embrace all emotions as felt – anger, displeasure, and grief to name a few. This is not to say that assertiveness cannot be friendly – it may or may not be. Indeed, attributes may be combined or may be exhibited independently. (The issue of "getting one's way" versus expressing thoughts and feelings is dealt with in detail in Chapter 5.)

Situations

The varieties of social exchange can be considered from two points of view – external and internal. The major external variable is the *other party* in the exchange. Internally, the child's *characterization of the circumstances* is important.

Other party

One child may well be able to say no to a sister but not to a friend; for another child, the reverse may be true.

Family. These are the people with whom children must live whether or not they like them or are liked by them. The consequences of social interactions cannot generally be escaped, so there are special constraints on behavior.

Peers. Some peers can be avoided but others (notably classmates) cannot. The emotional ties are not as great as with family, but on some issues – particularly for adolescents – friends/peers are a special influence.

Senior status. Authority must be reacted to differently. Being socially adept with the girl next door does not guarantee success with "big kids" or the teacher.

Junior status. Taking responsibility for others requires different skills from accepting authority. The call on leadership qualities is sometimes a function of a child's age, but it also reflects individual characteristics such as birth order in the family or popularity and sports ability at school.

Strangers. In mobile societies, strangers are a constant part of our lives. The greater the social difficulty presented by strangers, the more skillfully the child will avoid them – until contact is made inescapable by a major event such as moving to a new school.

Strangeness. Different demands are placed on a child's social resourcefulness by another type of stranger, not necessarily unknown as a person, but unpredictable in behavior: someone exhibiting strangeness, as with an unexpected psychotic episode or criminal intention.

Characterization of the circumstances

Not only does the other party influence social reaction, but overcoming embarrassment is different from communicating in the panic of a crisis.

Embarrassment. Sometimes we enter the wrong locker room and have to talk our way out of it. But most often embarrassment is *imposed* (by ourselves) on an otherwise neutral social exchange: joining in someone else's game, asking a person to dance.

Anger. Being angry and expressing anger are two different functions, especially with those we love or those we fear.

Fear. Ironically, the older children get, the more inept they become at expressing their anxieties. But at all ages children can be taught to overcome their fears.

Crisis. Skillful handling of everyday events is, to a point, an accurate predictor of reaction in a crisis. However, emergencies can have a quality that calls upon specialized social skills.

Processes

Whatever attributes are to be achieved in whatever situations, they will entail all the following processes to varying degrees.

Perception. First, we must see and hear the other person and interpret the mood, the message, and the "metamessage" (whatever is conveyed beyond the literal meaning of the words). For example, I might be a little depressed – the library computer search is still overdue – and I tell you it is okay to take the car tonight, but my tone of voice says you should never have asked. There is good empirical evidence that social ability is directly correlated with the speed and accuracy of recognizing facial expressions, among other things (see Trower, Bryant, & Argyle, 1978). Furthermore, perception involves seeing and hearing oneself: self-awareness without self-consciousness.

Cognition. Mediating between perception and response are thinking processes, which include making decisions, formulating goals, and anticipating consequences. These skills can be taught directly, as can cognitions appropriate to dealing with interruption or failure (see Chapter 5).

Judgement. A more global mediating process involves a comprehension of the larger situation – appreciation of culture, subculture, and personality. Our social reactions are considerably modified in the presence of a different ethnic group, a street gang versus a House of Lords subcommittee, or a specific individual. Such appreciations allow judgements of timing and an appraisal of relevance, in the face of the cultural and personal context.

Verbal communication. Overt processes in social exchange consist, first, of linguistic elements: words. The primary concern is with content: what is said and how it is structured.

Nonverbal communication. Second, overt processes are also nonverbal. This term refers to nonlinguistic elements: eye gaze, facial expression, bodily posture, for example. Less obviously, the form of speech (as opposed to speech content) is deemed nonverbal: voice characteristics, diction, hesitations. Some of the most interesting research in the nonverbal aspects of social interaction has been concerned with interruptions to conversation (e.g., West & Zimmerman, 1982). Even the mode of dress communicates in a social context and should be considered in building the repertoire of social skills.

For a more extensive list of verbal and nonverbal components see Table 1.1.

DEVELOPMENT OF SOCIAL SKILLS

Responsive tendencies to social encounter probably begin before birth with genetic endowment and differential growth of various parts of the brain. For example, hemispherical asymmetries of the cerebral cortex, clearly associated with language processing, have developed by birth (Galaburda, LeMay, Kemper, & Geschwind, 1978). (Given the plasticity of the brain – the ability of different parts to take over the functions of others – it is hard to interpret the implications of these anatomical differences.) Table 1.2 summarizes developmental characteristics, from the womb to puberty, that have relevance to social functioning.

A variety of social differences are apparent very early in infancy. It is recorded that at 3 months babies' heart rates slow down when they

TABLE 1.1
Specific Skill Components

Nonverbal Component	Adaptive	Extremes
face	expressive	exaggerated/blank
eye gaze	mutual	staring/averted
posture	relaxed	stiff/slumped
orientation	centered	towards/away
responsiveness	amiable	excessive/lacking
gestures	expressive	distracting/absent
voice volume	firm	shout/whisper
voice clarity	clear	clipped/mumbled
voice pitch	varied	exaggerated/monotone
pace	varied	too fast/hesitant
hesitation	allows thought	none/stumbles
handing over	engaging	too often/never
Verbal Component	Adaptive	Extremes
amount of speech	moderate	long/short
form of speech	articulate	verbose/garbled
sequences	linked	abrupt/unvaried
information content	interesting	unbelievable/boring
emotional content	stimulating	hysterical/lacking
expressiveness	suitable	excessive/absent

Sample observation scoring sheet in Appendix A.
Adapted from materials developed by Gaye Maxwell, University of Otago, Dunedin, New Zealand.

see themselves in a mirror, but speed up at the sight of another baby. Moreover, there are already gender differences: in the presence of peers, girls smile and gurgle more, whereas boys squirm more (Field, 1979). Within the first 12 months, there is ample evidence that humans need no special encouragement to engage in social interaction. Mutual gaze, greetings, and separation protests are well established. Researchers and mothers claim to be able to classify interactions as "friendly," "competitive," or "mean." Babies of that age make demands and denials and they imitate others (cited by Eckerman & Stein, 1982). The early ability to imitate implies a conceptual differentiation between self and others not predicted by Piagetian developmental theory. An amusing story has been related about a psychologist who had been studying early infant imitation some years ago. She was so excited by her discoveries that she went to considerable trouble to visit Piaget himself, she not think-

TABLE 1.2

Development of Social Functioning—Major Milestones

Age	Function
Prebirth	Genetic transmission of familial abilities
	Anatomical development of Broca's, Wernicke's and other areas of the brain serving speech
3 Months	Recognition of self in mirror
	Imitation of parent's facial expressions
	Gender differences in social response to peers
	Mutual gaze
12 Months	Greetings
	Separation protests
	Friendly vs. competitive interactions
	Complex imitations
2 Years	Gestures, two-word sentences
	Companion preferences
	Fear of strangers
	Cooperative play, including sharing, turn taking
	Aggression
3 Years	Sentences
	Substantial persuasion, including demands and protests
	Reciprocation of withdrawal and aggression
5 Years	Following verbal instruction, game rules
	Group functioning
	Boasting and other social ascendance
	Sense of fairness, guilt
	Talking to adults
	Seeking peers for play
7 Years	Imitation of older children
	Extensive seeking of praise, confirmation from adults
	Attachment to schoolteacher
	Anticipation of (specific) future events
9 Years	Formal cooperation ability, marked increase in listening
	Increased competition
	Manipulation or denigration of others
	Identification of a "best friend"
	Abstraction in language
11 Years	Ability to take other's perspective
	Formation of abstract concepts
	Imagination of futures and of alternatives
	Completion of linguistic and cognitive abilities necessary for social interaction

ing that he would not want to know. She told him that she had poked
out her tongue at infants only 3 months old, and how did he think they
had responded?

"They poked out their tongues, too!" she cried in her excitement.
"What do you think of that?"

Piaget was quiet for a moment before he replied: "I think that's very
rude."

It is now established that infants will mimic tongue protrusion and
a range of other facial expressions as early as 17 days after birth (Field,
Woodson, Greenberg, & Cohen, 1982).

During the second year, communication develops very rapidly. Gestures and two-word sentences are used to ask questions. Cooperative
play, which is spontaneous, creative, and includes turn taking, occurs
with others, as does aggression with apparent intention to hurt. The
child also becomes increasingly discriminatory towards social partners,
from mothers, fathers, and peers to strangers (Eckerman & Stein, 1982).

After the age of 2 years, toddlers begin to have genuinely verbal conversations with each other. The ability to make effective demands and
protests is well established by that age, but it is not until the third year
that subtleties of sustained persuasiveness appear (Ross, Lollis, & Elliott, 1982). Social deficits become reciprocated: children who withdraw
are left out, or in a sense, withdrawn from (Rinn & Markle, 1979); aggressive children are responded to with aggression (Patterson, 1982).
Therefore, it is not surprising that the major patterns of interaction of
3-year-olds tend to persist as if they were personality traits. The patterns of withdrawal and aggression are largely maintained by the reactions of others, and are therefore best thought of as behavioral disorders, as dealt with in Chapters 3 and 5.

By kindergarten, children have increased their ability to cooperate
and even execute short plans in small groups. But they also become increasingly competitive, with, for example, boasting and attempts to
usurp another's turn or share. Before long there is talk of fairness.

In the first year of elementary school, all forms of exchange from
sympathy to quarrels rapidly increase. An awareness of "growing up"
is manifest: older children are imitated, praise is constantly sought,
teacher's word is pitted against parent's, social events are greatly anticipated but may be dismally attended. After a year, positive attributes
of longer listening span and more group participation are juxtaposed
with episodes of taunts, bossiness, and extreme lack of grace in defeat.
Most children of this age have a "best friend," but more than one study
has found 10% of children to have no friend in their class and another

10% with only one friend (Van Hasselt, Hersen, Whitehill, & Bellack, 1979).

The rate of development of sophisticated language skills depends partly on the intelligence of the child but more particularly on the linguistic environment – how others speak to the child and what reading (or other language-oriented media) is encouraged. Between 4 and 8 years, communication for most children moves away from the predominantly nonverbal, with increases in abstract terminology and cognitive development. For example, "that one over there" becomes "the wonky one on top," and 6-year-olds will attempt to construct a story around random pictures (Stone & Church, 1984). Children also develop the ability to take the other person's perspective at times (Piaget, 1965).

For the average child at puberty, there are no linguistic or cognitive development barriers to being socially adroit in most situations. When children do not have social skills commensurate with their age, one of three possible reasons may apply: naivety – the skills have never been learned; inappropriateness – the skills are misapplied; or anxiety – the skills have been inhibited by nasty experiences.

CONSEQUENCES OF POOR SOCIAL SKILLS

As mentioned before, socially adept children have the chance of more fun. This assertion does not imply that enjoyment is necessarily the product of social interaction. If we were to define operationally "having more fun," we would attempt to measure as accurately as possible positive mood and other psychological functioning. Those with the greatest sense of euphoria and the least evidence of psychopathology would be deemed having more fun. But since enjoyment is such a subjective matter, it is appropriate to include another aspect to the definition – choice. If a child plays by herself when there are other children around, and does so by *choice*, not out of intimidation, then presumably she is having more fun by herself. Social skills often provide that kind of choice. The flip side of the coin is that socially inept children have less choice, resulting in diminished opportunity for fun.

That some children exercise less choice by virtue of less skill is a logical consequence of the definitions of social skill, as outlined earlier in this chapter. That these same children are less happy is a matter of empirical record. The evidence from studies summarized below is compelling. A multitude of disorders throughout the lifespan correlate with social deficits in childhood. Patterns appear to start early and to persist. In many of the correlations cited (at least those measured in the short term), the childhood deficit is implicated as the causal variable. The glimmer of optimism lies in the fact that, even when poor patterns have become established, new social skills can be learned.

Early Consequences

The two most conspicuous social deficits, withdrawal and aggression, are the most persistent. This phenomenon is understandable in view of the theories of reciprocity, which appear to apply in each case. Studies of toddler interactions (Rinn & Markle, 1979) indicate that when Ronnie is turned off by Jessie, Jessie is turned off by Ronnie. Thus Ronnie's withdrawal from peers tends to spread and to be maintained by all parties. A similar set of forces has been extensively reported on by Patterson (extensively summarized in 1982) in the maintenance of aggression in what he calls *coercive families.* That is, when children and parents try to control each other with negative sanctions (nagging before the fact, reprimands or spanking after the fact), the coercion tends to escalate – threats to verbal abuse to violence – and to be reciprocated. (Patterson's work is dealt with in some detail in Chapters 5 and 6.)

Aggression by peers is seldom reacted to adaptively amongst young children. Most typical responses are either retaliation in kind, or "I'm telling on you," neither case offering evidence of peer skills. Furthermore, in neither case is there real opportunity for development of the social repertoire. Support for the reciprocation theories is found in the longitudinal evidence that major social patterns recorded for 3-year-olds persist, if there is no intervention, through childhood, adolescence, and into adulthood (Hops, 1983).

These patterns may begin for a variety of reasons, the most common of which includes early family experiences. Harlow's (1958) studies with monkeys indicate that early isolation (within the first 6 months) leads to *either* shyness or aggressiveness. In adulthood, these monkeys fail as lovers and as mothers. But with monkeys or humans the disorder is behavioral, not a personality trait malfunction. The behavioral patterns may persist, however, because of a vicious cycle. Trower, Bryant, and Argyle (1978) have claimed that few people relate well outside their social strata. They point to the syllogism that we learn social skills from those around us, but the worse our skills the narrower becomes our circle, therefore the fewer skills we learn. . . .

School Achievement

Cartledge and Milburn (1978) claim that evidence for the impact of social behavior on academic success provides the strongest support for social skills training programs. However, the social behaviors in question are better described as "classroom survival skills" (Hops & Cobb, 1973). Mostly they center around interactions with the teacher: "attending" and "compliance" have generally been found to be the best predictors of academic success, as measured by reading and arithmetic achievement test scores. Systematic reinforcement of this narrow set of social skills has resulted in academic improvements, implying a cause and effect relationship. The reverse cause and effect is also claimed, but studies reporting the impact of reading tuition on social skills have been less than systematic.

School achievement also correlates with a child's ability to get along with peers. McConnell and associates (1984) rated reading achievement as the most important factor in school adjustment, and "negative initiations received" as the third factor of importance. More generally, it is found that peer interaction skills predict overall school grades and dropout rates (Hops, 1982).

Major stressful events, for example, loss of a parent (Kazdin, 1979), frequently have a severe impact on peer relationships and success at school. The trauma leads to lack of engagement with the environment, while other school-age boys and girls and the curriculum go marching on. It is regrettable that too often the gap is never bridged, or so it is implied by the overrepresentation of these cases among psychopathology in adulthood.

Adult Correlations

Many studies claim correlations between poor social skills in childhood and psychological disturbances in adulthood. It should be restated, however, that the claims are correlational. Many problems arise in trying to determine causal relationships between events over long periods of time. Not only are there the practical difficulties of keeping track of people in a mobile society, but there is the ethical necessity not to withhold the best possible treatment for unreasonable durations. There are no longitudinal studies that have treated social deficits in childhood to demonstrate an impact on adult disorders in contrast to control subject conditions.

Cowen and others (1973) documented the progress of subjects for 11 years. Children in the third grade were assessed on the basis of IQ, grades, achievement tests, attendance at school, teaching ratings, and peer ratings. The last proved to be the best predictor of adult mental health status. For example, children rated as the "bad guy" were two-and-a-half times as likely as other children to be on a community mental health register 11 years later.

According to Trower and others (1978), an inability in 10- to 11-year-old boys to see the other person's point of view is related to later delinquency. Hartup (1979) claims that moral development is a product of the quality – e.g., leadership, respect – not the amount, of peer contact received. Teenagers abuse drugs when both peers and significant adults abuse chemicals in like style – even if it is simply reaching for the aspirin bottle for every bodily ailment. (Delinquency issues are dealt with in depth in Chapter 10.)

Hartup makes extensive claims for effects of early rejection or isolation upon adult functioning. For example, adult sex crimes and also bad conduct discharge from military service both apparently correlate with childhood rejection or isolation. He also claims a correlation with mental hospital admissions. Trower claims that psychiatric outpatients show a high incidence (25%) of social inadequacy. This correlation is particularly high among men outpatients, of whom fully one-half are "socially inadequate" by Trower's definition.

Schizophrenic disorders in particular have social deficit precursors. Kazdin (1979) notes that childhood friendships, adolescent dating, and social activity all correlate negatively with *pre*schizophrenic behavior. In adulthood there are two outstanding correlates of schizophrenic relapse: one is neglecting the medication, the other is returning to a family with high "expressed emotion" (Vaughn & Leff, 1976). Expressed emotion refers to outspoken hostility and negative statements by relatives – a characteristic pattern that could change only with improved social responses on the part of the client. (Liberman and other authors – see Part I of Curran and Monti, 1982 – have developed extensive social skills training programs especially for this purpose.)

CONCLUSION

The previous discussions suggest the usefulness of early intervention in social deficits. There appears to be a good case for substantial benefit to lifetime patterns and the need to take action in early childhood. Academic success in school, itself a major influence on psychological functioning, seems to be influenced by a variety of social skills. The repercussions for adult personality, from childhood social deficits or strengths, are only tentatively understood, but the possible implications from correlational studies are enormous. In the next chapter strategies for skill training will be examined in overview.

CHAPTER 2

Approaches to Skill Training

Most techniques used to train skills for social survival ultimately involve the child as an active participant in the skill to be learned. That is, a major thrust of any intervention derives from activities which engage the child in coping with the difficult situations in question. Even with interventions that emphasize instruction, observation, or secondary (e.g., emotional) issues, participation in the skill activity is required sooner or later. Very often the situation is an analog – for example, a role play with other trainees. Techniques vary, essentially, according to the kinds of skills identified and to the processes that lead to engagement in appropriate skill activity. The issues of skill identification (*assessment*) and processes (*principles of change*) are dealt with in more detail later in this chapter. A plan for the general *components* needed to run a group program (since that has general applicability to the rest of the book), is then set out. Finally, the chapter addresses methods of gaining *cooperation*: with parents, significant others, and with the children themselves.

OVERVIEW OF TECHNIQUES

There is a vast array of different skills-training programs in use. Generally speaking, the more comprehensive the program, the better it works. To perceive an overview of the field, it is useful to conceptualize

19

programs as belonging to different categories. In broad clinical terms, three major classifications stand out: humanistic/psychodynamic, cognitive, and behavioral.

Humanistic (e.g., client-centered) approaches, *Gestalt* therapy, *Adlerian* therapy, and modern *psychoanalysis* have their roots in the psychodynamics of Freudian theory. What they practice in common are indirect techniques to address psychological problems, offering either insight or a "release" of pent-up disturbances.

Such techniques as play or art therapy (Schaeffer & O'Connor, 1983) or general group therapy (Yalom, 1970), or pure unconditional positive regard (Rogers, 1961) are sometimes used to treat social inadequacies. The most important contributions of these techniques are to the recognition and expression of emotions and to the development of the sense of self-worth. Elements of these procedures, acknowledged or not, are generally incorporated into other techniques. Most social skills training programs, as reported in the literature and as described in this book, are more direct. Important humanistic elements of therapy or training are described in the section "Rapport with the Child" (p. 36) and the psychodynamics of play and fantasy therapies are incorporated into different sections throughout the book.

Cognitive procedures include problem solving (Spivack & Shure, 1974) and self-statement training (Meichenbaum, 1977). Whereas both these techniques (described at length in Chapter 5) help children to develop their own reasonable plans and goals for an anticipated social exchange, they otherwise serve quite different purposes. Problem solving focuses on developing the ability to consider alternatives before the fact, whereas self-statement training prepares the child for self-control during the event.

By far the most commonly reported social skills training procedures are *behavioral*. Hops (1983) has suggested that procedurally this category can be further subdivided into contingency management, modeling, and coaching (which includes instruction, further modeling, rehearsal, and verbal feedback). Although this division is useful, it leaves a few gaps: for example, systematic desensitization (Wolpe, 1983), living environments (Risley & Twardosz, 1976), and videotraining (see Chapter 11).

A few years ago, Van Hasselt et al. (1979) pointed to the evidence for great promise of social skills training for children on the basis of overall efficacy of programs. At the same time, these authors pointed out the lack of evidence for which individual components within programs contributed to their efficacy – a state of the art that remains much unchanged today. The effectiveness of a social skills intervention depends on its comprehensiveness, its format, and its curriculum.

Comprehensiveness

Given that the most effective training packages are those with many components, it is valuable to examine the *types* of components that may be included. Any trainer's resources are limited, and the arbitrary addition of procedures will produce an unbalanced, unwieldy product. By contrast, an economically comprehensive package can be tailored by considering contributions on two dimensions.

On one dimension are three modes of behavior change. The term *mode* refers to the way in which learning or change takes place. The *vicarious* mode includes all that can be learned from observing someone else. It includes direct instruction and bibliotherapy, in addition to the more obvious format of vicarious learning by peer modeling (see Bandura, 1977b). In all cases, this mode provides examples of adaptive functioning that the client might emulate, if not imitate. In the second mode, the trainer provides consequation for the client specifically in connection with social behavior. That is, planful consequences are applied to alter future behavior, as in reinforcement, punishment, or extinction (cf. operant training, Skinner, 1953). The consequential mode is to be distinguished from the *experiential* mode in which the social behavior takes place in circumstances in which consequences *cannot* be controlled by the trainer. The experience itself may be anticipated to strengthen the skill (as with repetitive practice), or it may invite some predictable, natural consequences, which are, nevertheless, not controlled by the trainer. Modes may be combined, and frequently are in the most effective of strategies. For example, a child may overcome his fear of dogs through participant modeling, in which he observes someone approach and play with a dog (vicarious mode), then tries to approximate the approach himself (experiential), and is rewarded for successful approximations with praise and prizes (consequential).

The other dimension concerns the *medium* of the intervention; that is, the form in which the mode takes place. There are three mediums (I use that form of plural deliberately to avoid the connotations of media news reporting): imaginal, representational, and actual (live). Each mode can occur in any medium (e.g., covert modeling, filmed modeling, modeling *in vivo* are examples of the vicarious mode in each of the three mediums). Each medium has its distinct advantages and drawbacks that can be used to provide a balance of comprehensiveness and economy.

The *imaginal* medium has the advantage of low cost and lack of constraint. To have people do their therapy or training in their own heads avoids all costs of equipment, location, and extra personnel. It also allows scenes to take place that might not be possible otherwise; we can all surpass our real performances in our imaginations. However, some people have poor and fragile powers of imagination. The ability to visualize is highly variable, although it can be trained to some extent (Lazarus, 1977). Not all those with power to visualize may be able to control it very well. For example, a child may try to imagine her visit to the head teacher. The covert rehearsal may proceed adaptively when suddenly the imagined teacher becomes aggressive, the child starts to stutter, and the disaster worsens. These failures can be minimized with appropriate instruction, but another drawback remains. The major criticism of covert training is that the effects are weak relative to overt training (Kazdin, 1982). The guideline, therefore, is to use the imaginal medium when other methods are not possible or not cost-effective. These circumstances are by no means rare, so in many cases this medium offers the only route to therapeutic gain (Cautela & Baron, 1977; Wolpe, 1983).

The *representational* medium falls between pure imagination and real enactment. It includes audio and videotapes, books, films, and oral instruction, but stops short of play, even when the latter is symbolic. This medium has in common with the imaginal version its relative physical passivity for the client or trainee. Representation has the advantage, however, in that it does not rely on the trainee's imagery, either for its existence or for its accuracy. It is also distinctly the more powerful of the two mediums, if all other factors are equal. For example, if we show on videotape a child successfully joining a cliquey group of classmates, the effect will be considerably greater than if the child simply imagines it – provided that the same classmates are involved and that the social skills are equally fluent and effective. Thus the disadvantage of the representational medium lies in the trouble and cost of producing convincing and client-relevant materials, such as the example above of a child joining a specific in-group. Nonetheless, the trade-off between compromise and efficacy is such that even gross approximations are often effective. Perhaps the trainee's imagination can bridge the gap in accuracy, but remains, generally, controlled by the representation. Therefore, the representational medium becomes the treatment of choice when the effects through imagery for any reason are poor and when approximations to real enactments are not obtainable in sufficient quality or frequency.

The *actual* or live medium is potentially the most powerful, and, therefore, the medium to be given first consideration. Its distinguishing feature is that it involves the trainee in physical engagement, with at least analogies or approximations of personal effectiveness or, better still, actual engagement with the real thing. The potential efficacy must be weighed against the cost (including difficulty and time factors), and consideration should be given to combinations of approaches.

Mediums can be combined in two ways. The first is to make enough progress in one to proceed to a more difficult medium. This succession of approaches is used routinely in some interventions. For example, in the treatment of school phobias by systematic desensitization, children are typically required to deal with going to school, being at school, and interacting with others in a series of graduated approximations. Most usually, these situations are mastered first in the imagination, then *in vivo* (Wolpe, 1983). This process can be greatly speeded up by use of the representational medium (see Dowrick, 1983a). The other combinational approach is to take a hard-earned positive example of training and put it into an easier medium for frequent use. For instance, after half an hour's coaching to achieve a humorous reply to being teased by a sibling, the result may be captured on videotape for frequent review or it may be recalled from memory. Or a specially tailored first-person story may be remembered for repetitive rumination. Table 2.1 sets out a variety of common interventions falling within the different modes and mediums.

Format

The second major set of considerations affecting the impact of a social skills training program concerns who to involve, how often, and how long. Very loosely speaking, more is better. Studies so far have shown that no matter what type of approach is used, the most effective interventions are those in which training takes place frequently and con-

TABLE 2.1
Examples of Common Interventions by Mode and Medium

Medium	Mode		
	Vicarious	*Consequential*	*Experiential*
Imaginal	covert modeling	covert conditioning	mental rehearsal
Representational	filmed modeling	video feedback	self-modeling
Actual (live)	live demonstration	token economy	physical practice

tinues for a long time (Hops, 1983). Meeting once, twice, or three times a week keeps up the momentum. Session length depends on the comfortable attention span of the child or children involved, the attention span in turn depending mostly on maturity factors. With groups, less than one hour is usually too short a time to make progress, whereas after two hours boredom and fatigue become problems. In working with individuals, those time parameters may be halved. Crash courses of a weekend or a week do not allow reasonable opportunity to consolidate skills or to permit naturally occurring events to contribute to development. Most successful courses run 6 to 12 weeks, often supplemented with refreshers and advanced training.

The most complex aspect of format revolves around who to involve — individuals on their own, peers, or family.

Individuals. Training should be offered on a one-to-one basis willingly and conscientiously, but only when a group setting is inadvisable. It is not just the cost factor, it is that social skills cannot, by definition, be done in isolation. Nonetheless, certain conditions make it preferable to work individually. The most obvious case is that of a child who is so withdrawn that attempts to persuade him or her to join a group would result in outright failure or in poor attendance at sessions. Under such circumstances, individual training could be aimed at developing trust and collaboration as part of skills to participate in a broader setting.

Other cases arise from scheduling difficulties or other organizational problems, such as insufficient numbers of similar clients. However, group participation should not be ruled out too easily on the grounds of dissimilarity between individuals. Group functioning is often enhanced by some heterogeneity of skills and deficits amongst the participating children (see following section). The question remains where to draw the line. My tentative rule, given no research on the issue, is to form moderately heterogeneous groups. Ideally, each member will have something to offer at least one of the other children. At worst, the most deficient member will be within "learning distance" of the others. The coined term *learning distance* indicates an estimate that within the training period the weakest member of the group will overlap the abilities of some of the others. If available clientele are too diverse for this rule, then individual training would seem advisable.

The techniques most suitable to individual intervention for social deficits are systematic desensitization (Chapter 4), self-instruction training (Chapter 5), contingency management (Chapter 6), and self-modeling (Chapter 11). Elements of confrontation are valuable, as is repetitive practice. Individual respect (unconditional positive regard) for the person independent of behavior, always has a place, being particularly important in building rapport and trust.

Peer groups. Current evidence suggests that first consideration should be given to training groups of children with reasonably similar capabilities and goals. Increasingly available materials are being produced based on this concept. It is not simply the issue of cost benefit, but some training formats are suitable only for multiple clients. Some social skills training proponents have argued for the importance of group homogeneity (e.g., Kelly, 1985). However, as stated earlier, I have found that a reasonable variety of clientele and problems is not only tolerable but enhances the functioning of the group. There is a greater opportunity for children to learn from one another, which is generally beneficial both to the child who is learning and to the child who is seen by the others on a particular occasion as being an expert.

With a group, a reporting structure is available, providing support, reinforcement, and powerful stimulus control. It also enables vicarious learning and group problem-solving to take place.

Family groups. Possibly the movement of the future for training in some types of social skills lies in family involvement. Some of the most successful interventions with childhood aggression (Patterson, 1982) and juvenile delinquency (Alexander, Barton, Schiavo, & Parsons, 1976) have been family-based. (See Chapters 6 and 10 for social skills approaches to these issues involving multiple family members.) Social skills training for children without the involvement of their families sometimes has negative repercussions: assertiveness is mistaken for aggression, or other misunderstandings arise, with severe damage to newly acquired changes in the children's behavior. In situations where the targeted social interactions have particular consequence for other family members, the parents and siblings should, if possible, be involved. This strategy allows the goals of different family members to be reconciled, and for the complete system to adjust more uniformly. In most respects, the family group is similar to a peer group in format.

Curriculum

The final outstanding consideration for the impact of a program is its content. The first determinant of content is knowledge of the critical areas of deficit, methods for which are described in the next section. Once the deficits have been determined, it is crucial to identify exactly the skills necessary to overcome them. Whereas the general principles of instruction and training apply in nearly all situations of social competence, it is the detail of curriculum that bridges the gap from abstraction to practice. Thus subsequent chapters deal with certain procedures for shyness as distinct from aggression and others for emotional disturbance as distinct from physical handicap. This book is organized to provide details of curricula against a background of selected procedures.

ASSESSMENT OF DEFICITS

There are two purposes of assessment. One is to enable an evaluation of an intervention, a primary concern to researchers. The other is to guide the intervention itself, essential to practitioners, and the major focus of this section.

Whether for planning or evaluating an intervention, the assessment is concerned with social interactions. Social interaction assessment procedures tend to examine either the amount or the quality of interaction. Both aspects, determinations of which are seldom found in the same procedure, deserve attention. The quality of infrequent interaction, for example, distinguishes the genuinely isolated child from one who is highly independent. At the other end of the scale, the class bully may be classified amongst the most popular, if frequency of interaction was the sole criterion.

Choice of Assessment Procedure

In recent years there has been a proliferation of assessment instruments for socially unskilled children (Asher & Hymel, 1981; Cartledge & Milburn, 1980; Curran & Monti, 1982; Goldstein, Sprafkin, Gershaw, & Klein, 1980; Hops & Greenwood, 1981; Michelson, Sugai, Wood, & Kazdin, 1983). Even limiting the possible issues by age and current functioning level, there exist enough to spend more time on individual assessment than there is available for treatment. The goals of assessment, therefore, are 1) to limit the number of skills to be taught, 2) to identify those skills most crucial to survival or enhancement, and 3) to identify the skills most reasonably amenable to change. That is, the assessment procedure should be manageable, at the same time providing information of value to the immediate intervention. Standardized assessment instruments, where available, are useful to research, but they frequently need modification to serve a specific population (cf. Wallander, Curran, & Myers, 1983). Different assessment approaches are discussed relevant to various social deficits in subsequent chapters, and sample forms are provided in appendices.

The total number of itemized social skills, from catching someone's eye to maintaining friendship in the face of jealous misunderstanding, would fill a volume of fine print the length of this book. In practice this list is limited by the following strategies. It may be assumed that all major nonverbal communication patterns (see p. 11) will be trained or verified in training. For the purposes of *intervention* planning, therefore, these skills need not be assessed separately from the more complex skills pertinent to the population. Furthermore, the search for deficits may be limited to those most relevant to the age group or to any special purpose of the training program (e.g., reducing delinquency). Due appreciation of the importance of developmental levels is often overlooked in child therapy (e.g., children are not miniature adults [Harris & Ferrari, 1983]; see list of major developmental milestones, p. 12).

To identify those skills from which the child will derive most benefit, a checklist should be developed with two scales: ability and benefit. Teacher or supervisor ratings are most useful, except for those circumstances in which the presence of an authority figure interferes with the social interaction. Therefore, subject self-ratings should also be used for family, boyfriend or girlfriend relationships, and interactions with other authority figures (e.g., police).

For research it may be appropriate to use standardized role play, with videotape and observers, in addition to behavioral checklists (see examples in Chapter 5). However, role play has some drawbacks. Clients tend to role-play what they think is socially desirable, not necessarily their usual behavior, and ability to role-play varies greatly. Standard role plays are useful, but their limitations must be borne in mind. In practice, role-play assessments most frequently can be achieved informally during early sessions. It is used mostly to verify the subjective report measures.

These assessment strategies should be used to find three or four skills of major importance for each individual: for example, accepting a compliment, saying no to drug pushers, asking to join in a card game. The total list thus generated for the group can be reduced further by considering skills of greatest potential impact. Initially, we identify two or three that are common to several clients, and fairly easy to learn. These are to be taught first, at the same time incorporating nonverbal skills that emerge as needing to be trained. We then identify one or two other skills per client, to be taught later with more individual attention. Equal time should be allocated to each child.

The preintervention assessment is thus manageable. It provides, at low cost, a program of intervention with the right number of target skills (one or two per session), including those both beneficial and accessible to the clientele. With the addition of "consumer satisfaction" questions, the same assessment procedure can be used after intervention to provide some program evaluation, necessary to the integrity of any childcare or therapy. (See Table 2.2 for an example of an assessment strategy.)

Assessment, however, is not confined to before and after testing. It is an ongoing exercise. Pretesting allows the development of an intervention plan, which, all being well, may be largely adhered to. But the plan should be flexible. Observational assessment by the trainer should continue each session, with constant revision being considered. Very often skills take more time and practice than may originally be budgeted for. Occasionally events during the course of training quite alter the value of the curriculum.

PRINCIPLES OF CHANGE

Our knowledge of techniques to facilitate learning is being expanded and refined. Certain theoretical viewpoints (e.g., operant conditioning theory, Piagetian developmental stages) suggest specific learning strategies and response classes to identify in the children we work with. Nonetheless, a number of *empirically* proven approaches to training exist, regardless of theoretical orientation. It seems valuable to summarize them here. All the techniques identified are valuable to any program, but some are especially suited to certain conditions. Therefore, more detail is provided in subsequent chapters.

Information

Every skill has associated with it a body of information: the circumstances in which a certain reaction may be called upon, the elemental components of skill performance, the probable effects following the action or the consequences of not reacting. There is always some value in the intellectual appreciation of such facts. Learning is assisted by an understanding of what is to be learned. Subsequent generalization of the skill to a variety of circumstances may be enhanced by further information. Most training sessions, therefore, begin with an educational component. The trick is to provide enough relevant information to be useful without tedium, and without the misunderstanding that an in-

TABLE 2.2
Example to Illustrate Assessment Strategy

1) *Group identified*: developmentally disabled teenagers. Plan for standard group intervention.
2) *Impressionistic concerns*: immature reactions to personnel in work settings being trained for; embarrassments with peers of opposite sex.
3) *Specific examples*: supervising personnel report walkouts following criticism and anger outbursts with workmates; teenagers report not knowing how to respond when others touch them.
4) *Data collection*: no standardized procedures available seem suitable for this specific population, therefore adapt one from another setting. A self-report checklist is used (see Appendix E) that includes items such as, "Do you find it difficult to ask for a favor or anything else from a supervisor?", "Do you find it difficult talking to someone of the opposite sex?", and a range of other issues. Each of the 20 items is rated on a 5-point scale of difficulty. Twenty further ratings are similarly given to items that are identical except that they ask for the *importance* to the client rather than the difficulty.
5) *Client input*: the trainer goes over all the questions in 4) with each youth, a time-consuming but important process with this clientele. Each youth is also asked the open-ended question, "Are there any other social situations that bother you?" Questions are used flexibly (providing notes relevant to individual circumstances) to discover the real issues, not to be bound by formality.
6) *Other opinion*: for each client, the same forms are responded to by a supervisor.
7) *Consolidation*: three items per client are identified as being most difficult and most important for him or her. Any sharp discrepancies by supervisors are added to the list (in this case, difficulty in telling someone off, and difficulty in standing up to someone who is pushy).
8) *Common priorities*: three skills are noted as most common to the youths, and not of advanced difficulty. (In this example: saying something in a group; asking a favor of the supervisor; seeking information from a doctor.)
9) *Individual priorities*: more difficult issues for individuals are noted; for example, being criticized by a specific female supervisor, and taking a job interview were issues important enough to two individuals that time might be spent on them.
10) *Intervention modification*: curriculum of the planned intervention for the middle and final sessions is adapted to reflect the assessments. Early sessions for initial training of this population (see Chapter 9) inevitably focus on nonverbal expressiveness and receptiveness. Middle sessions incorporate items from 8) above, one issue per session, adapting the issue for each client in turn. Final sessions incorporate issues from 9), one issue per session, focusing entirely on the individual concerned with other group members in support.
11) *Ongoing assessment*: intervention remains flexible to new information, in-session role plays, and other observations. Curriculum must wait until skills curently being taught are well learned.
12) *Post-assessment*: checklists are readministered to clients and supervisors after intervention is complete, and again three months and six months later. Youths and their supervisors are also asked to rate consumer statisfaction questions, such as, "Do you think what you learned in the course helped you get along better in the workshop?"

tellectual appreciation can substitute for action. This balance is easily achieved by setting time limits. Talking about issues, what to do, and why, should always comprise *less* than one quarter of the time spent in training. Following this guideline forces a trainer to become suitably economical with the educational component.

Information may be provided in a number of different forms. Direct instruction ("in these circumstances, if you do this, such and such will happen") has its place, added to which some less obvious methods are particularly useful with children. Asking questions leads to more engagement, telling stories can be memorable, audio and videotapes are more graphic. The use of puppets often provides the best of all worlds for young children.

Modeling

The most rapid method of teaching a new skill is to demonstrate it — that is, to provide a model. Even when the technique works imperfectly in and of itself, it serves as a valuable prerequisite to other procedures. Modeling is the ultimate description of how to perform a skill. For these reasons, modeling is used early in the training session, in a natural sequence following information. Bandura (1969) claims that most social behaviors are learned in normal settings by observing similar behavior in others. Therefore, it is logical to use this observational learning process deliberately in the remedial setting.

However, most of the skills in the training curriculum will have been previously observed somewhere (other children, adults, television), and it may be asked what the conditions of modeling are that give it efficacy. There are many ways to give modeling poignancy. One is the focus provided by including the specific social interchange in the training program. Other means center around two factors: the appreciation of the payoffs — the *usefulness* of the behavior; and the ability to identify with the behavior of the actor — the *meaningfulness* to the observer. Therefore, it is valuable, for example, to show the positive change in attitude that results from a firm voice and pleasant smile, for example, rather than to demonstrate the behavior without its consequences. The meaningfulness to the observer can be enhanced by being realistic about the child's level of sophistication (models who are seen to struggle a little at first — not instant experts), and by using a model who is not unlike the observing child behaviorally and in other ways (allowing identification with the model). The principles of modeling, or vicarious learning, are given some detail in Chapter 3.

Rehearsal

The step immediately following an understanding and observation of a new skill is trying to do it. Rehearsal then is the experiential phase following the vicarious phase. For most social skills, only a very weak form of learning will take place without physical practice.

Rehearsal also provides circumstances for rewards and other feedback. Furthermore, a good rehearsal offers an ideal model for another trainee.

Conditioning

The main principles of conditioning are reinforcement, punishment, and extinction. (Studied in the laboratory and in the field, their application to social interaction is dealt with most extensively in Chapter 6.) In brief, rehearsal and verbal report allow opportunity for praise and other differential reinforcement to strengthen adaptive responding and to eliminate interfering behavior.

It is a common misunderstanding that conditioning is manipulative. In fact, it helps the child develop control rather than imposing control on the child. Instead of conceiving reinforcement as "controlling" the child – a terminology that suggests the child is powerless – it is more useful to characterize the child as "seeking" reinforcement. Systematic application of conditioning principles can enable the child to discover a variety of means to obtain the sought reinforcements and to appreciate some of the costs or benefits that inevitably accompany social actions in this complex world. In this sense, the child is provided with choice, through which intrinsic rewards and self-reinforcement will inevitably emerge.

Correspondence

What young children say they do is generally disparate from what they actually do. The accuracy of verbal report is referred to as *correspondence* (Risley & Hart, 1968). The correspondence between saying and doing, while inexact at any age, is a developmentally dependent response class; that is, the disparity decreases as the child grows up. The development of correspondence can be greatly speeded up by simple intervention. When appropriate feedback is provided, children tend to alter what they do to match what they say. For example, suppose a child is capable of telling her father what normal courtesies are, states her intentions to exercise them, but then forgets. Her lapses are not likely poor memory or deceit. If her discrepancies are systematically pointed out to her (as detailed in Chapter 9), she is more likely to knock before entering, say "please" and "excuse me," rather than to alter what she says about what she does.

Feedforward

Behavior is guided both through past experiences and by future anticipations. Feedback provides information about past (usually recent) performances; *feedforward* is a term coined to refer to information about future performances (Dowrick, 1983b). An understanding of this principle helps to clarify why positive reinforcement works more reliably than punishment and why modeling works when the client can identify with the role. In practice, feedforward requires a focus on those skills or skill components that can adaptively be used more often in the future. Effective feedforward often defines apparently new skills that are attainable by enhancement or recombination of existing component abilities. Feedforward ignores past errors (see Chapter 11).

It is interesting to observe that modeling, conditioning, and correspondence training all embody the feedforward principle: each in its own way *defines* the behavior adaptive to future functioning. Modeling illustrates it in someone else's actions, conditioning pinpoints its components in the existing repertoire, and correspondence training prompts what is understood into action. These ideas will be more readily appreciated after the relevant procedures have been examined in detail.

Cognitions

In recent years there has been renewed interest in the relationship between thought and behavior. Most particularly it has been recognized that maladaptive thought patterns can induce anxiety or maintain depression, thereby contributing to a lack of engagement in social activities. It is useful during training sessions, therefore, to pick up on these interferences whether they are explicit (maybe verbalized as "I'm no good with girls") or implicit (e.g., recognizable from excessive hesitation with a well-practiced skill). Interfering cognitions can be systematically replaced with thoughts that facilitate action (see Chapter 5). It may be noted, however, that it is not cost-effective to spend session time examining what children think about what they do, except when troubleshooting a specific impasse. Even then, the emphasis is on training the coping cognitions, rather than exploring details of the interference.

Environment

Every social exchange is different because the environment is forever changing. This circumstance makes adaptation more difficult unless we learn how to structure the environment to our advantage. *Environment*, as the term is used here, includes every aspect of a person's context: internal states, other people, and physical surroundings. Complex skills can be taught by providing a very safe environment initially and gradually increasing the level of difficulty or of threat. Systematic desensitization for the treatment of fear (Wolpe, 1983; see Chapter 4) is the most well-known approach that uses this strategy. However, the principle can be incorporated into all training. Skill acquisition is more enjoyable, and generalization is enhanced by providing a variety of contexts – imagination, role play, and reality – and by starting with the least demanding tasks and proceeding in a hierarchy.

Assignments

Only a very few environments can be created within a training setting. Just as it is important to translate an intellectual understanding into practice, so is it essential to transfer a skill rehearsed in a sheltered environment to a real-world situation. Thus every session should end with the delineation of assignments (referred to in many programs as homework) to be met before the next meeting. Assignments that involve only observation (e.g., watching television with the sound off to observe nonverbal communication) are safe and therefore useful early in training, but are limited in value as learning experiences. As clients progress, assignments that allow practice involving a small element of risk can be chosen; for example, saying hello to the new girl in the classroom. It is necessary, of course, to predict the most likely reactions of other parties involved to minimize the chance of a negative experience.

Group Work

The virtue of training in groups goes beyond the advantage of having an assortment of peers with whom to interact. The group provides support. The trainer can set an example, and if necessary, insist upon group members being positive and supportive towards individuals in the program. The support is a social skill in itself, but will come with suitable prompting in the context. Encouragement from peers is often the most powerful reinforcer available. Also the group provides a reporting structure for assignments and for other social events of relevance that occur between meetings. One element not necessarily evident from research published in journals is the potential to have fun in social skills training groups.

Esteem Building

The building of social skills and self-esteem with children is a leapfrog affair. The development of one is synergistically related to the other. Social skills programs are usually not systematic in the enhancement of self-esteem. The weight of the evidence suggests that social success leads to a child feeling good about himself, more than the other way around. However, self-belief enables perseverance in the face of adversity, as suggested by Bandura's (1977a) concept of self-efficacy. It may be that the basis for confidence and determination is independently as well as incidentally trainable. Therefore, training strategies specific to self-esteem are elaborated in Chapter 8.

GROUP TRAINING COMPONENTS

Below is a summary of the major considerations in planning and running a group social skills training program.

Assessment

Measure: Checklist scored by child and supervisor/parent
Choice: Depends on age and "problem" of group
Targets: Determine maximum three per child
Choice: Most relevant and most amenable for group
Reduce list of target skills to 1-2 per session
Goals: Set individually with and for each child

Composition of the Group

Number of children: 6-10
Range of deficits: Mildly heterogeneous
Trainers: Preferably two (male and female)

Meetings

Frequency: 1-3 times per week
Length: 1-2 hours
Course duration: 3-12 weeks

Session Format

Review previous assignments
Information and scene setting:
    Descriptions, vignettes, role play, role reversal
Solutions:
    Brainstorming, modeling, problem solving
Practice:
    Rehearsal, cognitions, expressiveness, relaxation
Feedback:
    Reinforcement, error correction
Feedforward:
    Clarification, self-modeling, reassurance
Assignments:
    Individual minigoals, self-assignments, generalization

Program Format

First session: Overview of the course; familiarization
    with each other, goals and concepts, video; personal rights
Early sessions: General skills (e.g., recognizing
    feelings, asking open-ended questions), basic to many
    interactions; additional emphasis on nonverbal components
Middle sessions: Specific target skills common to several
    group members (e.g., dealing with taunts about being
    overweight)
Closing sessions: Highly individual problems or complex
    skills (e.g., making conversation with the only girl in the
    world who makes this child so embarrassed he can't
    think)

COOPERATION OF PARENTS AND OTHERS

The attitudes and behavior of family, teachers, or anyone who extensively interacts with a child will seriously affect the progress of training. Occasionally children need to be trained to survive their environment, whatever it is. But most often the environment can and should be altered to facilitate the change. The following guidelines will prove useful.

1) For each child make a list of two or three individuals who have the most impact on the child's daily life (by virtue of authority or proximity).

2) Inform them about the program, emphasizing its educational nature and its benefits to all concerned.
3) Involve them in some aspect of the program. Possibilities include: assessment, assignments, progress reports.
4) Listen to their opinions, particularly specific examples of their observations. Modify the program to fit family and school circumstances.
5) Solicit general support with specific ideas on how they can arrange circumstances conducive to change and how they can respond appropriately to facilitate change.
6) Be available for comments and questions at any time.

RAPPORT WITH THE CHILD

Throughout all phases of the program, much of its success will depend on the trainer's social skill with the children. A good rapport is not in itself a sufficient condition for success, but it is almost always a prerequisite. Most professionals preparing to set up a social skills training program already will have worked extensively with children and will have many of the prerequisite abilities. Provided here is a checklist of reminders in the art of building rapport.

Body Language

Be prepared, frequently, to get down to the child's height – look at them at their eye level.

Most children, but not all, like to be touched.

Face

Children appreciate more expressiveness – particularly smiles – than adults do.

Exaggerated expressions (amazement, pretending to cry) amuse children, helping them to laugh and to relax.

Vocabulary

Simplify your language, as appropriate for the developmental level, but remember that children's comprehension exceeds their expressive capacity. Therefore, use language that is a little more sophisticated than their vocabulary and syntax.

Good News

Express appreciation whenever possible, particularly nonverbally.

Bad News

Reprimand only when it is necessary to change a child's behavior. Then a verbal explanation must be given in terms of behavior (not personal worth), and time must be taken to teach the change in behavior.

Attention

Listen and make the level of attention clear when a child talks. If the child interrupts it is better to propose talking later than to give half attention.

Follow through on promises; the child may be too shy to reinitiate.

"I" Statements

Children, no less than adults, do not benefit from being told what they think or feel. But they do gain from being told how others feel as a result of their actions. For example, a teacher might say "I feel exasperated when you mumble and won't look at me," rather than "You always think the teacher's out to get you."

Statements such as the latter are like trait labels (e.g., "you clumsy oaf"), which can also be avoided with "I" statements ("I can't talk while you're bumping into things"). Note that in most cases, "I" statements include what might be called behavior statements: " . . . when you mumble . . . while you're bumping into things . . . "

"You" Questions

Children more than adults can benefit from an expressive guess of how they feel. For example, a child seems depressed. It might be appropriate to say: "I've been thinking about your dog dying. Are you feeling depressed about that?" It is important to be careful about second-guessing another's feelings, however, even with young children. Avoid assumptions in the place of questions. Note that even "Are you depressed because your dog died?" provides an *assumption* that the child is depressed.

Other Questions

The use of more questions than statements helps to keep children engaged. It also gives them more sense of contribution and self-assurance.

Nonverbal Communication

Just as the trainer must teach it, the trainer should exercise it. Even with children who are poor at expressing their feelings, an observant trainer may still read the signs.

Respect

Because of the power vested in adults and because of the discipline problems of children in some settings, it is difficult on occasion not to lecture or to patronize. Avoid language that would be inappropriate if addressed to an adult (e.g., "Don't be a wimp," – unless said with humor). Respect shown will become mutual.

CHAPTER 3

The Shy Child

Shyness is the problem most commonly associated with social skills deficits. It is characterized by the void left by nonexistent skills, not by maladaptive behavior patterns in their place – as in the case of aggression. Indeed, isolation or social withdrawal is the condition most frequently addressed by the literature on social skills training with children. Major reviews (e.g., Conger & Keane, 1981; Hops, 1982) and books (e.g., Zimbardo, 1977) have been devoted to the topic.

This chapter describes the manifestations and implications of shyness, and also how isolation may be assessed. The most successful procedures for helping the shy child are then presented, followed by a case study for illustration purposes.

THE NATURE OF SOCIAL WITHDRAWAL

The term *shy* is short and simple, which is why it was chosen for the title of this chapter. However, the word refers to what somebody *is*, suggesting a static quality, perhaps intractable to change. Moreover, we often hear of shyness used to explain paradoxical behavior: "He's only that boisterous because he's so shy, deep down inside." For the purposes of a skills-training program, it is better to act upon what we *see*; issues arising from children who are boisterous because they are shy will be dealt with in Chapter 5 on aggression.

39

The *isolated child* is a useful and frequently chosen term. It refers to the social condition in which a child finds him- or herself, and it thus provides a step towards meaningful identification of children needing help. But the most useful term is *social withdrawal* because it refers to what the child *does*. It refers to a *lack of self-expression or other participation in group events of a social nature*. It does not refer to a child's decision not to participate out of preference, however. When the lack of expressiveness or participation takes place because there are *no alternative skills in the child's repertoire*, then a training program can be of benefit.

Passivity

Children may withdraw from social interaction by failing to initiate, or by responding negatively when they are approached by someone else. A simple indicator, then, of social withdrawal is a count of the number of interactions made by a child in a social setting (e.g., school playground). Greenwood and associates (1977, 1979, 1982) have made a careful examination of *interaction rate and duration* as an indicator of social withdrawal. Their measure is based simply on the number and length of interactions, without regard to the nature of the interchange, and thus gives rise to a *consolidation score*, which is essentially the total time spent interacting in proportion to the time spent in company (Greenwood, Todd, Hops, & Walker, 1982).

When the consolidation score (quantity of interaction) is *very low*, it appears to have excellent validity. That is, children with very few interactions tend to be unpopular with peers, to be rated by teachers as friendless, and to avoid social initiations by classmates. This tendency is, of course, a generalization, and many special cases exist of passive children who maintain popularity.

Negativity

For children who exhibit a *moderate* amount of interaction, the *quality* of the exchange becomes more important. For example, it is evident that a child may isolate him- or herself by virtue of introducing a socially negative tone in response to friendly overtures by other children. However, the empirical findings of observational research indicate that the quality of exchange is less important than might be expected. For the kindergarten through third-grade children in Greenwood's study, negative responses occurred at a rate of only 6% amongst the most highly interactive children, and even less among the other children.

Reciprocation

Lack of initiation in social contact appears to be the single most important variable in social withdrawal. The shy child's response to another's contact is also important, but less so. Compared with the average child (statistically average in amount of interaction), the isolated child makes one-third as many initiations, and receives one-half as many. Nearly all the shy child's initiations are received without rejection but do not increase without specifically supportive intervention.

Therefore, the objectives of an intervention should be:

1) to expand the range of approaches a child might make to another;
2) to improve the ability to maintain engagement.

Frequency

It is claimed in surveys (Van Hasselt et al., 1979) that amongst young school-age children, 10% have no friend in their class, and another 10% have only one. It is probably conservative to estimate that *one-fifth of all children* are isolated enough to benefit considerably from a social skills intervention with the above objectives.

Long-term Consequences

Social isolation tends to increase rather than decrease with the passage of time. The pattern exacerbates itself, and there are claims that peer rejection is an enduring condition by the age of 9 years (Oden, 1980), or even by 3 years (Hops, 1982). Lack of popularity correlates with school dropout (Roff, Sells, & Golden, 1972) and other academic problems. There is also some evidence for social isolation as a predictor of adult emotional disturbance (Cowen, Pederson, Babigian, Izzo, & Trost, 1973; Kohn, 1977; Roff & Hasazi, 1977) and psychopathology (Kazdin, 1979). The evidence is sparse, however, and indicates more variable and less serious long-term consequences than for other social disorders (at least aggression; Conger & Keane, 1981).

ASSESSMENT

Shy children, by their very nature, are easily overlooked. Therefore, assessment may be required in two different circumstances: screening or intervention planning. For example, a teacher working with an arbitrary mixture of children may wish to identify (screen) those children isolated enough to require special attention. Or a childcare worker may have a group of children already identified, and therefore would need to assess the nature of their social deficits to design an appropriate intervention.

Screening

Competent teachers or supervisors sufficiently familiar with the group of children to be screened are well placed to make the initial assessments themselves. This provides the least costly approach.

In some cases entirely unstructured methods have been used. That is, teachers have simply identified the "most isolated" children in their classes (e.g., Evers & Schwarz, 1973; O'Connor, 1969). Given the research data cited earlier, one might expect to identify five or six children in every class of 30 without undue alarm. A better method that greatly reduces the potential for unintended bias and provides more information is a standardized checklist. A good example is the Walker Problem Behavior Identification Checklist (WPBIC, Appendix B; Walker, 1970). It provides a measure of "Withdrawal" to be compared with other children of the same age. It can also provide scores on other measures (e.g., "Distractibility"), and can be completed in a short time.

An alternative method of assessment, referred to as a *sociometric rating*, is more suitable for supervisors less familiar with their clients. This method rates children according to peer acceptance. In its simplest form of administration, it requires every child in the class or group to name, for example, three classmates they especially like. The total number of nominations received is then a measure of popularity, and children with two nominations or fewer should be given further assessment. It should be noted that a sociometric rating measures a different phenomenon from a supervisor rating. The child's popularity is a ranking relative to others in the group, and as such reflects a complex set of social interactions. Very young children can be asked to point to photographs, rather than make written replies (see Asher, Singleton, Tinsley, & Hymel, 1979).

Variations on the sociometric ratings include asking questions such as, "Who do you like best to work with?" These measures are more reliable when all children are rated (on a 5-point rating scale, say) by all others in the group, rather than by each child making a small number of nominations. Some researchers (notably Asher & Hymel, 1981) have argued against behavioral observations in favor of sociometric ratings as valid measures of social withdrawal. However, it seems that one type of measure is not to be pitted against the other. Sociometric ratings are invaluable for screening; behavioral observations are indispensable for intervention.

Intervention Planning

Considerable gains can be made with interventions that target total interaction duration, without respect to the nature of the interactions (Greenwood et al., 1982; Hops et al., 1979). However, given the important differences in social norms on the basis of age, gender, and subculture, a more explicit assessment is highly desirable. Most screening assessments are designed only to identify those most at risk for the disorder or deficit in question and should be followed up with a more explicit consideration. None of the above procedures are ideal for pinpointing skills most necessary to be worked with. The WPBIC is moderately helpful, but even that instrument only samples the behaviors to be targeted.

More specific information is necessary for meaningful intervention. Behavioral observations used in studies are elaborate and tedious, necessary for research and publication, but not used for interventions except occasionally with individuals. In group training for social withdrawal, curricula are often preconceived, sometimes "on the basis of the literature," and sometimes, it seems, even more intuitively. Rather than abandon direct observational assessment altogether as a basis for planning interventions, a compromise is necessary.

In some cases, shy children are referred for treatment. In these cases, informal observations are already available as the basis of referral. Although informal, these observations provide a valuable beginning. Referred cases often present extreme social dysfunctions, and systematic observations are then warranted, as in the case study described at the end of this chapter. Other cases, however, are easily overlooked, because of the background nature of social withdrawal. Thus the screening procedures described above are necessary to identify those children at risk on the basis of isolation or unpopularity. Because neither of these conditions assures that the problem is social withdrawal, further observations are necessary. Various sources, such as published checklists (e.g., the WPBIC) and anecdotal data of those who supervise the children, will help.

Ultimately, the observations of the intervention planner are essential, possibly incorporating a specially devised response form that keeps the task simple, but provides sufficient focus on aspects relevant to the age group, the setting, and other population characteristics. Such assessment can necessarily be developed only by the social skills trainer in a specific setting over a period of time. The assessment procedures for apparently aggressive children, described in Chapter 5 ("Troubleshooter for the Social Jungle," pp. 80–82), may serve as a model for this purpose.

INTERVENTION STRATEGIES

Vicarious Learning

Most learning of social behavior takes place vicariously (Bandura, 1969, 1977b). That is, we learn a lot simply by observing others. Even when observation by itself is insufficient for behavior change, it powerfully facilitates subsequent learning or learning by other means. Expressed loosely, observation provides information about what we potentially could learn. Therefore, it is most appropriate that the vicarious learning strategy is the first to be discussed in detail. Whereas vicarious learning takes place in natural settings, the discussion below refers to planned demonstrations from role plays, whether by children or adults, sometimes on film or videotape.

Other terms for vicarious learning include *observational learning, modeling,* and *imitation.* These terms will be used interchangeably unless a distinction is necessary. Observational learning may be defined as "the behavioral change that results from the observation of others engaged in similar behaviors" (cf. Bandura, 1969, pp. 118–119). According to Bandura, four mechanisms are involved: attention, mediational encoding, motoric reproduction, and motivation. That is, our sensory faculties must first track the observable behavior, the brain then stores the information in memory, we must subsequently be capable physically of producing our own version of the behavior, and finally we must be prompted with the circumstances to put the learning into action.

Withdrawn children do a lot of observing. But they do very little observational learning of social skills. It seems that these children may attend quite well to the relevant interactions of others and possess the motoric reproduction capabilities, but their deficits are critical in other areas. Therefore, a vicarious learning training program needs to make certain aspects of behavior relevant and salient to socially withdrawn children and to provide evidence of positive outcome.

Salience. Major methods to make observed social interactions meaningful include the use of multiple models, similar models, various situations, and verbal discussion. The use of multiple models simply implies that it is better to have three actors than one. Preferably the actors would be diverse, suggesting that these skills can be achieved by all sorts of children. Diversity improves the chances that an observing child will find one of the actors to be similar to him- or herself. The identification with the model, which overcomes the interfering thought of "it's all very well for that person" may be of critical importance to shy children. Most particularly, the similarity should be behavioral. That is, the best models will be those who have the appearance of shyness and are seen to overcome it—referred to as coping models as opposed to mastery models. In an interesting study with preschoolers, Jakibchuk and Smeriglio (1976) compared first-person to third-person narration on videotapes of children overcoming their problems of social isolation. It was found that a first-person admission to shyness was critically more valuable in the induction of a modeling effect for the observing children.

Presenting a variety of situations provides a sense that these skills are not specialized, and thus facilitates generalization. Verbal discussion of what the models were doing improves the child's memory of the observed events. It also helps generalization and discriminating use of the skills, based on the perspectives of others in the training program.

Outcome. Shy children may be well aware of how to approach other children, to initiate conversation, and to maintain an interchange. They may also be capable of performing the repertoire. But they may be very unsure of or timorous about the outcome.

A modeling procedure, therefore, should focus on the skill, its context, *and* its consequences. The outcome must demonstrate clear intrinsic benefits to the initiator. This vicarious reinforcement will provide a source of motivation for the trainee when a suitable situation presents itself.

Modeling Procedure Example

O'Connor (1969, 1972) performed some classic interventions with shy preschool children, thus providing good examples of filmed modeling with more than a modicum of experimental control. The basic procedure was to show isolate children a film of their peers in social interaction. The film of 23 minutes presented scenes in a sequence that "systematically graduate[d] the activity level and the number of children engaged in the interaction" (O'Connor, 1972, p. 329). It had a sound track adding descriptive information to elaborate both the action and the outcome; in this respect, it provided possibly critical salience to the vicarious learning experience.

The children in these studies were selected from several preschool and nursery school classrooms. Teachers first identified a sample of their children as the most withdrawn by their own judgement. Then these nominated subjects were observed and selected on a criterion of exhibiting fewer than 5 out of 32 predetermined social interactions. In the 1969 study, nearly half of the subjects were lost because of their own shyness: some were frequently absent and others refused to go to the film room. Six children completed the intervention, four girls and two boys. Two of the children increased the frequency of their interactions dramatically from about 3 to 25 as measured, while the others made enough improvements to bring the group's average number of interactions up to the average of nonisolate children that had been randomly chosen from the same classrooms. For control purposes, a comparable group of isolate children were shown a film about dolphins and they showed no change in their withdrawal.

O'Connor confirmed these results in his later study (1972), with a greater number of children. He also compared the effects of the film with the effects of reinforcement (trained graduate students giving praise and attention), both by itself and in conjunction with the modeling film. Surprisingly, the reinforcement factor made no measurable difference. This finding was essentially confirmed by Evers and Schwarz (1973) who used the same film and teacher praise for attempted reinforcement. By contrast, Walker and Hops (1973), also using O'Connor's film, but with primary-grade children, demonstrated that token reinforcements, carefully applied, can serve to sustain and enhance the initial effects of the film. First they determined the relative initiation rate between the isolate child and her peers. If the isolate child's rate was high, *she* was rewarded for approaches toward her by her peers; if the isolate child's rate was low, her *peers* were rewarded for initiations by the identified child towards them. When both rates were extremely low, both contingencies were applied, and this was found to have the most powerful effect of all.

These external reinforcements can be made to occur only after the child has attempted the modeled skill. The natural reinforcement (e.g., the success of positive interaction), and with it the most compelling understanding of outcome, can be achieved only through actual experience. Thus most so-called vicarious learning programs include an experiential component (cf. participant modeling, Bandura, 1969). (Aspects of experiential learning will be discussed in more detail in the next chapter.)

Social Environment

A related aspect of considerable relevance to shy children is the construction of a social environment that is particularly conducive to engagement subsequent to modeling. Two principles in particular deserve attention. One is to ensure that the environment provides opportunities for social engagement. The other is to provide positive outcomes for any attempt to interact. Different methods of using children's peers to create engaging and rewarding social environments are described in an edited volume by Phillip Strain (1981).

Example

One of the most thoroughly developed programs for shy children is the product of an extensive research program at the Center at Oregon for Research in the Behavioral Education of the Handicapped (CORBEH) by Greenwood, Hops, Walker, and colleagues. Their program, called PEERS, comprehensively includes instruction, demonstration, and reinforcement, and, as the acronym suggests, it emphasizes the involvement of same-age, nonisolate children. (For a thorough description, see Hops, Walker, & Greenwood, 1979.)

The children for whom this program was developed were primarily in preschool and early grade school. They were identified as socially withdrawn on the basis of a global measure of interaction time. Under this system, children are observed in recess or other free-play periods in which their total social interaction time is directly estimated on the basis of a structured sampling procedure. (See discussion of consolidation score, p. 40) Because younger children generally spend less time in social interaction, the researchers developed norms for different age groups.

The objectives of the PEERS program are to provide collaborative play and academic activities for the isolate children, to encourage their peers to assist the collaborations, and to teach specific skills of interaction. These objectives are met by the four major procedural components discussed below.

Social skills tutoring. Each identified child meets with a selected peer and a trainer for 15-minute tutoring sessions. Typically there will be five sessions over the course of a week. The child is first guided in ways to initiate talking or playing with another child. He or she is then taught how to maintain interaction, with specific attention to praising and cooperating with peers.

Reinforced play. Each day during recess the child is encouraged to put the tutored skills into practice. The child is offered points for interacting with others. Three or four peers are assigned (from volunteers) to facilitate earning the points, which later contribute to a reward for the whole class.

Academic collaboration. Each day during class, a task requiring turn taking and verbal interaction is assigned to the child and a peer. To begin, the tasks are highly structured (e.g., responding to flash cards); later they may be more spontaneous (e.g., discussing a painting). A different peer is found each time to facilitate generalization.

Correspondence training. Before recess the child is asked, "What are you going to do during playtime?" Immediately after recess the child is asked to report back with the assistance of a special helper. This reporting structure produces a correspondence between what the children say they plan to do and what they actually do subsequently (Risley & Hart, 1968). (Correspondence training is discussed in more detail in the context of developmentally disabled children in Chapter 9.)

The PEERS program is appealing because of its general applicability and because a teacher can be trained by CORBEH in two days to implement the procedures. The program appears to be very effective for the most withdrawn children — about 2 to 5 out of 30 — in typical classrooms for the early grades or nursery school. However, it does not address specific deficits that may be important to specific children (although program development along these lines is currently underway [see Finch & Hops, 1983]). Other considerations in the use of peers in social skills training are touched on in Chapter 4.

The program examples selected to conclude this chapter, although giving less attention to structuring the environment, illustrate more specifically tailored approaches in the group setting and on an individual basis.

A GROUP PROGRAM FOR PRIMARY GRADES

A comprehensive group-training program for shy children has been described by La Greca and Santogrossi (1980). This program fits quite well into the *general paradigm* described in Chapter 2. It was developed for *third- through fifth-grade* children with moderate social deficits – a slightly older group than those around which the PEERS program was developed.

Children were *selected* on the basis of sociometric scores. Classmates rated on two separate 5-point scales how much they liked 1) to play with and 2) to work with others in the class. Students less popular than the average on both scales were considered for participation. These measures correlated so highly with each other (.92) that for children of these ages it seems that only one scale, play or work, is necessary. It is also clear that the program included many children who were not severely isolated.

The effective *training procedure* was a 4-week program with weekly sessions for 1½ hours after school. The groups comprised five children – either all male or all female (an unexpected and unexplained allocation). There were two group leaders – one male and one female. At a preliminary meeting the purpose of the group was explained: "to learn better ways of playing and working with others." The children also were informed about what to expect in training; namely, videotapes of other children, discussions, and role play.

The *curriculum* for the program was devised on the basis of published knowledge concerning peer acceptance (e.g., Oden & Asher, 1977), rather than specific assessments of the children involved. However, the content was comprehensive, including the following components described in detail by La Greca and Mesibov (1979):

- smiling
- greeting
- joining others' activities
- making invitations
- conversing
- sharing and cooperating
- praising
- attending to physical appearance

In each of the four treatment sessions, two different skill areas were trained in a *set format*. First a 4-minute videotape was shown with peer models demonstrating the skill at issue. Three boys and three girls were seen in a variety of situations, each scene resulting in positive consequences.

The children then *discussed the tapes*: What were the other children doing? How could what they did be applied to their own daily interactions? Next the children *role-played* self-relevant situations (e.g., joining other children's games), practicing the skills identified on the videotapes. The trainers offered suggestions and made video recordings to use for *feedback* purposes. Children were encouraged to *critique* both positive and negative aspects of their own performances. However, this procedure has an element of danger, particularly for less competent children. It is generally unnecessary to draw attention to deficits: most benefit can be gained by soliciting positive and constructive comments only. (See Chapter 11 for a full discussion of these issues.)

Finally, children were given *assignments* (e.g., "Greet a classmate at least once a day for the next week"), which were reviewed at the beginning of the next session. With five children per group, and two assignments (or one double assignment) per child, it would be helpful to write down the assigned tasks at the end of each meeting.

The *results* reported for this program are generally impressive. The intervention program described above was compared (using equivalent groups of other children) with "attention placebo" and waiting-list control conditions. Before and after the intervention, in addition to the sociometric ratings mentioned, a variety of measures were taken, including skills knowledge, role play, and behavioral observation. In all these latter measures considerable improvements were found. The results are particularly noteworthy in view of the relative brevity of intervention. It is recommended in social skills training that a much greater number of sessions be planned.

The only measure not showing statistical significance was the sociometric rating of peer popularity. Whereas it may seem ironic that the screening factor was the least affected by treatment, it should first be pointed out that peer acceptance will change much more slowly than knowledge and skills. Second, a point overlooked in other discussions of this issue, a property of sociometric ratings is their self-adjusting relativity. That is, the ranked popularity of one child can increase only at the expense of another's. One cannot take the less popular half of the class and train them so that everyone is above average. Therefore, one may well train unpopular children to become more friendly, more accepted, and more socially skilled without significantly altering their ranking in a fixed group. In any ranking, raising the overall standard cannot change the fact that someone must come last: what is true of the Olympic Games is true of the classroom.

CASE STUDY WITH A PRESCHOOLER

Single case studies are presented throughout this book because of the tangibility of detail provided, and because children are sometimes too individual to be dealt with in a group setting. The case presented here involved Charles, a 4-year-old boy who was so shy that he would have been unable to take part in a group intervention. He was treated with self-modeling (Dowrick, 1983b), a procedure discussed in detail in Chapter 11 on videotraining.

Procedurally, self-modeling differs from peer modeling in that the trainee sees a videotape image of him- or herself, rather than that of another child. A powerful rationale for using this approach with Charles is provided by the results of the study by Jakibchuk and Smeriglio (1976), mentioned earlier (p. 45). The peer-modeling films they made for shy preschoolers were similar to those of O'Connor, except that the voice-overs were spoken by a child. They found the films to be far more effective when the child spoke the commentary in the first person, rather than the third. The procedure of using a first person child commentary appears to be an intermediate step between having a peer model on the film, and contriving to show the trainee him- or herself engaged in model behavior. The following procedure, used with Charles, was developed independently of this rationale at about the same time as the above study. (As written here, it is condensed from journal publication [Dowrick, 1979]).

The Shy Child

"Charles," at nearly 5 years old, was so shy he would scarcely speak to anyone except his mother, even in her presence or when spoken to by others. He was referred to me at a child psychiatric unit. In the course of systematic observations, we found that he could be persuaded to remain in a playroom without his mother, but he stayed close to the door and would not approach within 10 feet of other children in the room. He was judged to have no speech defects. His mother reported that Charles's father was also extremely reticent verbally, except when drunk – a comment that later proved surprisingly useful.

Videotaping

Three videotapes were made in the playroom. The first was made with judicious recording and editing to create the impression of Charles approaching a small group of other children. This effect was achieved by taking advantage of the apparent shortening of distance produced by the telescopic lens and by editing the best approximating behavior.

After watching this tape for 3 minutes only twice, Charles "imitated himself" by rapidly joining the other children in the playroom. However, he remained on the periphery most of the time, making occasional nonverbal interactions. Eventually, a self-model film was edited from recordings of these low-frequency interactions.

Before Charles was shown this self-model tape, however, his mother chanced to remark on her husband's garrulousness when, and only when, intoxicated. The psychiatrist then agreed to see if Charles would be similarly disinhibited with Valium (diazepam, 5 mg). Remarkably, within half an hour, Charles was chatting so fluently to a sandbox companion that a self-model "talking" tape was easily made.

Training

Charles attended the unit twice a week for 2 months. He first saw a self-model tape (3 minutes). For research reasons no comment was offered, but presumably selective praise may well have enhanced the effect. Charles then was given free time in the playroom with a potential peer playmate and observed through a one-way screen. No instructions were given to the peer and no incentives or rewards were offered to either child.

Observations recorded at each session were as follows:

1) the latency of Charles's approach to the other child who was placed in the activity setting (measured in seconds);
2) the frequency of nonverbal interactions defined as: eye contact, adding to the other child's play, reaching in front of the other child, or offering something to or taking something from the other child;
3) the number of words spoken.

As indicated in Figure 3.1, the three self-model films were shown to Charles in succession. After a baseline in which no film was shown (four sessions), the approach film was presented (three sessions), then the nonverbal interaction film (four sessions), and the verbal interaction film (six sessions).

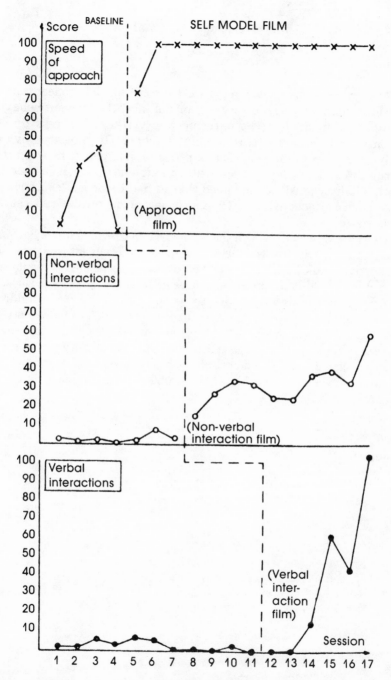

FIGURE 3.1. Observations of Charles's social interactions in multiple baseline analysis. (Note: speed of approach is calculated as 100 minus latency in seconds.) Reprinted from Dowrick (1979), with permission of publisher, Haworth Press.

Results

Observations are shown in Figure 3.1, from which it is clear that after one or two viewings of each self-model tape, the relevant behavior changed very rapidly. The outcome was verified a success by the parents, and Charles settled happily at school. His mother provided daily ratings from the home setting. In the final phase, he was rated at the top end of a 5-point scale for talkativeness, at which time his mother lightheartedly complained that he had become a "chatterbox." Telephone contacts 3, 6, and 12 months later confirmed his successful socialization.

This case was one in which the learned skills provided immediate and sustaining positive consequences. The social environment was generally supportive, and Charles obviously enjoyed the social engagement once he had mastered it. In many instances of social withdrawal with very young children, this may prove to be the case. With older children, however, more attention to generalization and maintenance may be necessary. It is also evident that Charles learned the appropriate social skills very rapidly, suggesting that a component of anxiety was at issue. In more extreme cases, when skills may be present, but overwhelmed by anxiety, we have children whose problem is not shyness, but fear.

CHAPTER 4

The Fearful Child

A fearful child differs from a very shy child by the *specificity* of the circumstances in which he or she becomes so withdrawn. A child who is afraid of all social interaction may simply be called shy, and the procedures in Chapter 3 are appropriate in dealing with the problem. However, some children may be socially adept in most circumstances, but phobically inept in others. It is less a question of nonexistent social skills, but more an extreme anxiety which swamps those abilities in a narrow set of situations. Specific social phobias must be identified, and treated differently from social withdrawal.

PHOBIAS OF PEOPLE AND INSTITUTIONS

Shyness occurs, typically, when skills are absent, and therefore new skills need to be taught. Fearful children, on the other hand, have skills that are inhibited in specific circumstances. Thus the task for the trainer or therapist is to disinhibit existing skills, rather than to establish new ones. Surprisingly, perhaps, *phobias*, as distinct from general shyness, have not been focused upon as an issue for social survival. The material in this chapter has been selected and adapted from findings and methods applied to all varieties of phobias.

Specific fears should be differentiated from general anxiety. When

children are nervous in a wide variety of circumstances, the condition
should be viewed as emotional disturbance, and given more comprehensive analysis and treatment. (The relationship between emotional disturbance and social functioning is examined in Chapter 8.) Morris and
Kratochwill (1983, p. 29) suggest seven criteria by which to identify
specific fears. A *phobia*

1) is out of proportion to demands of the situation;
2) cannot be explained or reasoned away;
3) is beyond voluntary control;
4) leads to avoidance of the feared situation;
5) persists over an extended period of time;
6) is unadaptive;
7) is not age- or stage-specific.

These criteria all support the severe maladaptive nontransitory nature of a phobia. However, a further criterion must be added to reflect
the specificity of a phobia which

8) is a characteristic reaction to a narrow set of circumstances.

Traditionally, much has been made of the *origins* of phobias. Witness
the famous and controversial descriptions of Sigmund Freud's Little
Hans and John B. Watson's Little Albert (Freud, 1909/1963; Watson
& Rayner, 1920). In Freud's case, Hans's phobia (of horses) was attrib-
uted to an Oedipal complex and fear of castration. The infant Albert
provided a demonstration by Watson that phobias (of furry animals)
could be acquired through classical conditioning. Unfortunately, much
of the energy put into the debate about the origins of fear appears to
have been wasted from the clinical standpoint. In perhaps 90% of cases,
phobias are successfully treated by attention to the fear problem as it
currently exists, with scant attention to the cause. Factors *maintaining*
the fear may be important but factors of origin are not. Most often, the
origin of a phobia is never uncovered. Whether or not a phobia has been
learned is not as important as the fact that it can be "unlearned."

From the biological standpoint there is some claim that humans are
predisposed to fear of certain aspects of the environment much more
readily than others. This predisposition has been termed *preparedness*
by Seligman (1971). Suppose a small boy has a very scary experience
in the dark at his back doorway, with his brother, after eating strawber-

ries. If he does develop a phobia as a consequence, it will most likely be a phobia of the dark, not of his brother, the doorway, or strawberries. Why the dark, of all possible stimulus events? It appears we are, with evolutionary connections, predisposed to acquire fear of some objects or events more readily than of others; darkness is one. A snake is another, height yet another.

Of all the common phobias (those with Greek prefixes, e.g., claustrophobia), only three are socially oriented: people (anthropophobia), being alone (menophobia), and strangers (xenophobia). This small number may reflect a bias of our evolutionary predispositions. Despite the tendencies and probabilities, phobias can develop with *any* object or event. With an increasingly complex society, disabling social fears are becoming more common and much more important.

Miller, Barrett, Hampe, and Noble (1972) make an interesting claim for three basic dimensions of childhood fear. These are physical injury (e.g., flying in an airplane), natural or supernatural events (e.g., thunder, ghosts), and social anxiety (e.g., reciting in class). The items they list in each category appear to depend for their classification on certain assumptions, however. For example, "being kidnapped" is listed under physical injury, whereas "being enclosed in a strange room" is a natural event, and "separation from parents" is a social anxiety. Despite their classification, fully one-third of all the listed fear situations are clearly and inextricably concerned with people and institutions. Miller and colleagues also claim that the tendency towards fears of natural and supernatural events diminishes with age, while the propensity in the other categories increases. In a thorough review of age factors in childhood fears, Graziano and Mooney (1984) revealed few and unsurprising differences "for so much research activity" (p. 91).

ASSESSMENT

A child is more often referred for help by a concerned adult, usually a parent or teacher. Under these circumstances it is essential to make some confirmatory, direct observations of the child in the situation of risk. It is neither necessary nor desirable to terrify the child to verify the concern. A gentle approximation of the situation will suffice. When the fear has been confirmed, it is valuable to assess its specificity and intensity, and how long it has been a problem. Further assessment depends on establishing the goals of intervention.

Specificity

Specificity should be established to rule out the possibility that the child is either withdrawn or emotionally disturbed and therefore in need of a different kind of treatment. If the child is withdrawn she or he will be reticent in a large number of social situations, because of an absence of the relevant skills. To rule out social withdrawal it is necessary, therefore, only to find evidence of these skills being applied in at least some circumstances. This objective is readily achieved by identifying situations with equivalent demands and observing how the child copes with them.

For example, suppose Janet is extremely fearful of small group activities in class, whereas she works well by herself. If she lacks the ability to take turns or to speak up for herself in the playground, with family, or in other settings, she has a skills deficit and is better treated as a shy child. But if she is unassertive only in the classroom setting, the possibility of phobia should be investigated further.

It is valuable to note the importance of early identification of problems. A specific phobia may develop from a general skills deficit after a period of time. In the above example, if Janet had been shyly unassertive in a class that demanded extensive group work, she may eventually develop a fear of going to school at all. At the same time, she may be quite happy going to Brownies. In this case, it would be necessary to treat the school phobia both for its anxiety component and for the skill deficit (lack of assertiveness). Thus, in any case of a recognized phobia, the possibility of attendant deficits should be investigated.

Sometimes a specific phobia is identified when a general anxiety is present. A suitable screening device is a self-report survey that includes items beyond social anxiety. Several are available that provide scores and norms—for example, Children's Manifest Anxiety Scale (Castenada, McCandless, & Palermo, 1956; revised by Reynolds & Richmond, 1978) and State-Trait Anxiety Inventory for Children (Spielberger, 1973).

Perhaps the most promising self-report survey for purposes here is the Fear Survey Schedule for Children, developed by Scherer and Nakamura in 1968 (described by Morris & Kratochwill, 1983, pp. 92–95). It contains a wide variety of potential fear items, including "going to the doctor," "getting a bee sting," "being teased," "nightmares," and "spiders." A modified version by Ryall and Dietiker (1979) contains only 50 items (the original contained 80), and uses a 3-point scale ("not scared or nervous or afraid," "a little scared," "very scared"). It is designed for children from kindergarten through sixth grade. (The complete survey is reprinted in Appendix C.)

Self-report measures have been sharply criticized for their limitations for research or intervention planning purposes (see Morris & Kratochwill, 1983). However, it is impractical to survey a broad range of situations expediently any other way. If a child shows up as "very scared" on several diverse items, it is better to put aside the intervention strategies described in this chapter and to refer the child on for clinical attention. Some kind of social skills training may be helpful (see Chapter 8), but probably as a supplement to another intervention.

Intensity and Duration

Once the specificity of the fear to a particular social setting is established, it is valuable to investigate its severity. Graziano and Mooney (1984) have suggested that a fear has clinical significance if it has an intensity that is debilitating to the lifestyle or has persisted for over 2 years. The purpose of the time frame is founded on the observation that children frequently "grow out of" even quite severe fears within this period (Hampe, Noble, Miller, & Barrett, 1973). However, 2 years is a large proportion of an 8-year-old's life; therefore, "debilitating to the lifestyle" may be more frequently applied.

Duration of a fear is simply established by asking the child or the parent – preferably both. Even if onset is quite recent, say a few weeks, help should be offered if the condition is intense. For our purposes, the intensity of the fear is the extent to which it disrupts the daily life, education, or development of the child. Thus, if the child is missing school, significant recreational activities, or otherwise missing out, he or she should be provided support. Such a judgement can be made jointly by the child and concerned adults.

Further assessment depends on the type of treatment chosen and is developed as part of the intervention. For research and evaluation, critical assessment tools are direct observation, self-monitoring, and psychophysiological measures. (These are extensively reviewed by Morris and Kratochwill, 1983.) Direct observation provides the most reliable measure of relevant behavior in all its aspects. Self-monitoring provides access to information not otherwise easily obtainable by others. Psychophysiology is valuable for its objectivity, and because strong fear reactions bring with them severe changes in physiology, some of which have considerable impact on health.

Goals

It is always clinically beneficial, and ethically desirable, to establish goals of treatment in collaboration with the client. Even when it is difficult – for example, with very young or disabled children – setting goals for treatment should be attempted to the extent possible (see Chapter 12 and Sheldon-Wildgen & Risley, 1982). With the fearful child, it is therapeutically more imperative than with other children needing social skills. As Barrios, Hartmann, and Shigetomi (1981, p. 269) have pointed out, fearful reactions of children (e.g., crying, running to a parent) are adaptive responses to genuinely threatening events. In colloquial terms, goal setting is the product of asking the questions: "What do you want to get out of this? What don't you want to give up? How, exactly, do you want to be, further down the line?" The art is to find an answer that is meaningful and unambiguous to all concerned.

Criteria for goals. A treatment goal describes the behavior of which the client will be capable if the intervention is successful. The description should be that specific for it to be unambiguous to all concerned. As an illustration, one of the treatment goals in the case study at the end of this chapter states: "By 6 weeks Scott would visit a doctor or a dentist and show no more apprehension than an average 5-year-old." This specification, as with any treatment or training goal, faces the following criteria:

1) *What behavior* – ("visit a doctor or a dentist") can be observed and recognized.
2) *Where it occurs* – in Scott's case this was considered, but thought unimportant, provided it was off his home territory.
3) *Frequency* – once was enough at 6 weeks.
4) *Magnitude* – ("and show no more apprehension than an average 5-year-old") implied it would be observed by people familiar with 5-year-olds.
5) *By when* – ("by 6 weeks") provides an understanding of the cost of treatment – emotional, physical, or financial.

An explicit goal specified in this manner is not a contract, however, such as those by which sales personnel earn their commission. But it provides a sense of direction and a satisfactory basis for review. It also allows subgoals to be formulated. Ultimately, the *implied* goal of intervention must be examined; the behavior change achieved is meaningful only if there results a subjective benefit to the child and those caring for the child (see "Changing Social Behavior" in Chapter 12).

INTERVENTION PROCEDURES

The interventions described in this chapter differ from those in other parts of the book in that they are more clinical and are generally not suitable for group implementation. Nor are they reflected in much of the social skills literature. However, these interventions address target areas essential to the social functioning of many children today. And elements of the procedures make a fundamental contribution to other interventions.

Experiential Learning

As thematically emphasized in Chapter 2, virtually all training packages contain an experiential component. For example, observational learning often requires participation by the trainee, practice of a new skill makes for perfection, and attempted repetition is necessary for training by successive approximations. It is also worth examining experiential learning in its own right. Simply engaging in a behavior improves the probability of doing it at another time.

Experiential learning refers to the changes of behavior, thought, and feeling that result from the experience of action. Examples include rehearsal, role play, response prevention, and graduated performance. Learning through experience does not imply that consequences (reinforcers) play no part in the learning, as Skinner (1938) and others would insist they do. But it is implied that the trainer exercises no control over the consequences – except perhaps to predict them. The trainer's role is to make verbal prompts: "Walk to the gate, look at the school, and walk home again every day this week," "No, you can't leave yet," and to plan the environment: for example, to arrange small work areas all in unobtrusive view of the supervisor. Learning takes place from the experience of the prompted actions and the environment (and their natural consequences).

The crucial relevance of experiential learning for the fearful child lies in the fact that phobias result in avoidance behavior that is self-perpetuating. For example, Larry is afraid of school. So Larry stops going to school. When he skips school, his anxiety is reduced – a very positive feeling, a feeling so positive, in fact, that it reinforces his avoidance. The only way this pattern can ever change is for him to experience school in ways more rewarding than avoiding it. That is, when he goes to school his anxiety does subside and other positive experiences (usually inevitable or natural, rather than trainer-controlled) reinforce his attendance. Simply put, he is able to discover from firsthand experience that school is not such a bad place after all.

Training that depends on experiential learning can succeed, therefore, only when the natural outcome of the action is rewarding, or at least benign. It is applied to social phobias only when the relevant social skills are established in the repertoire but inhibited in a narrow set of conditions.

Whereas there are numerous forms of experiential training in clinical child psychology, two subcategories make contributions of particular relevance to social skills of the fearful child. These strategies (described below) are graduated performances and the use of peers.

A brief mention is inserted here concerning *response prevention*. This term refers to strategies such as flooding, in which rather than removing an anxious child from a threatening environment, immediate avoidance is prevented (see Rimm & Masters, 1979 for a thorough description of flooding with adults; Smith & Sharpe, 1970 offer a rare example of response prevention with a childhood phobia). The essential feature, commonly overlooked, is that the anxiety *must subside* before the client leaves the situation (cf. getting back on a bicycle after a fall: one should stay on the bicycle until the jitters and tears have stopped). Although flooding has rapid results, it is seldom used with children. Rather, the less controversial techniques described in the following sections are favored.

Graduated Performances

The best known, perhaps prototypical, example of graduated performance procedures is *systematic desensitization*. Developed by Joseph Wolpe (1954, 1983) on a principle of reciprocal inhibition, it was presumed to work on the basis of reconditioning the feared stimulus. That is, it proceeded from the premise that one cannot be both anxious and relaxed at the same time; these are incompatible physiological responses. If one has a phobic response to a small furry animal (or a large hairy teacher), it was then assumed that, given proper training, one could condition in its place a relaxation response to that same animal (or the teacher).

Despite the logic of the original rationale, there is considerable debate over the underlying mechanism of systematic desensitization, although there is no doubt concerning the great efficacy of the technique (Kazdin & Wilcoxon, 1976). In practice, systematic desensitization proceeds through a large number of graduated performances, beginning with an object remotely connected to the phobia. At each step, intended to condition a relaxation response, the stimulus is made more similar to the feared object. It may be that the fine graduations of performances provide the most active component in the procedure. The treatment of school phobia described below exemplifies this procedure.

School Phobia Application

A case reported by Lazarus, Davison, and Polefka (1965) is interesting for its description of the basic systematic desensitization procedure and some enhancing variations. It seems that most studies reported in detail exhibit exceptions and innovations. The individuality of the cases and the lack of control conditions make it impossible to prove that any such variations were strictly necessary. However, they were implemented on the basis of clinical judgement and served to make the procedure more enjoyable and engaging to the client.

Lazarus and colleagues treated a 9-year-old boy, "Paul" after three weeks of his refusing to attend school. The process is set out under headings that may be generally applied to systematic desensitization.

Assessment and goals. Considerable background data, in particular family history and prior school experiences, were collected in Paul's case. He had suffered a number of emotionally and physically disturbing (even life-threatening) experiences in his nine years. He had refused to attend school once previously because of an intimidating teacher, a situation that was ultimately solved by a school transfer. On the other hand, Paul had had some very positive school experiences. Lazarus and colleagues concluded that "Paul's school phobia was the most disruptive response pattern of a generally bewildered and intimidated child" (p. 226). They made the clinical judgement that the primary objective of therapy was to reestablish school attendance.

The goals for school phobia are very straightforward. They were not reported in the article, but very likely could have been expressed as: short-term, 3 months – Paul, unaccompanied by therapist or parent, will attend school for the whole school day, each day for a week uninterrupted, without specific material incentives; long-term, 12 months –

Paul will maintain attendance as good as or better than the average of his classmates, not including any instance of medically verifiable illness. Ethical considerations suggest that these goals would have been developed collaboratively and agreed upon by therapist, Paul, and at least one parent.

Developing a hierarchy. Having established current, nonanxious performance (skipping school altogether) and the final goal (regular attendance), the next step was to develop a series of graduated, intermediate goals called a *hierarchy*. Hierarchies are usually established first in a small number of broad obvious steps (less than 10), which are subsequently refined into a large number of small steps that enhance and regulate the flow of progress. Complete hierarchies are often in the order of 100 items long (see examples in Rimm & Masters, 1979; Walker, Hedberg, Clement, & Wright, 1981). The broad steps in the program by Lazarus et al. were:

1) Walk from house to school.
2) Visit school after hours.
3) Attend school for first session, accompanied by therapist.
4) Attend school all day with therapist in classroom.
5) Therapist not in classroom, but in adjoining library.
6) Therapist leaves school one hour before closing.
7) Therapist at school half a day.
8) Paul attends school alone, earning specific rewards.
9) *Goal*: Attend school unaccompanied and without reward.

(This 9-point hierarchy was not developed by Lazarus, but has been derived, for illustration purposes, from an examination of the published report.)

The steps appear to be approximately evenly spaced, according to what is commonly referred to as *subjective units of discomfort* (SUDs). It is valuable to attempt an equal spacing, but not to be bound by it. As many items as necessary are added as intermediate steps; whenever the transition is found to be too great, more can be added. In the Lazarus application, a large number of small transitions were necessary around what are listed as items 6 and 7 above. A means of developing a basic hierarchy is set out in Table 4.1.

The countercondition. Lazarus trained Paul in relaxation and emotive imagery. The latter refers to the deliberate imagining of pleasant events such as a visit to Disneyland or receiving a much-prized gift. Relaxa-

TABLE 4.1

A Suitable Method of Constructing a Basic 9-Point Hierarchy

1) Establish a highly specific treatment *goal* from the initial assessment procedures. This goal is item 9 on the basic hierarchy.
2) *Brainstorm* a list of 15 or 20 situations that provide any degree of discomfort between baseline (current performance) and the treatment goal. Include a range of items from very mildly to quite severely disturbing. Vary them according to *theme* (talking to classmates may be thematically different from sitting in class) and according to *time or distance* (first session vs. whole day; two blocks vs. front door).
3) Identify the situation *closest* to baseline as item 1. Then consider which one is *about halfway* between baseline and the goal. Make this situation item 5.
4) Find the situation that seems to be *halfway*, on the dimension of difficulty, between items 5 and 9. This is item 7. Determine item 3, the midpoint between items 1 and 5, similarly.
5) Repeat the bisection procedure to establish all even-numbered items, midway between the points so far determined.
6) The above procedure establishes a first approximation to a 9-point hierarchy. Examine the intervals of discomfort between adjacent items. Where the intervals seem to be unequal, items can be replaced or further items added (the number 9 is not sacred, notwithstanding Chinese folklore).
7) The hierarchy can then be expanded simply by adding more steps between items. Usually a hierarchy is expanded at least two- or threefold before treatment begins. During treatment further expansion may be made as necessary.

tion and emotive imagery are good examples of responses incompatible with anxiety. Whether or not these incompatible responses are *essential* to training is debatable, but it is clear that pleasant physical and cognitive alternatives *enhance* the procedure considerably. Relaxation training is most common, and some time is usually spent on it as a prerequisite to further therapy.

Methods of relaxation training developed for adults (e.g., Rimm & Masters, 1979) should be supplemented with special considerations for children. For example, Frederick (1980), working with 10-year-olds, recommends guiding children to discover elements of muscle relaxation in their own terms. He uses humor: "Today we will have a brief lesson on 'How to do nothing'"; and many questions: "Can you make your heart stop beating?" Finally, he guides their discovery: "What did my face tell you when it was relaxed?" Students reply, "Nothing," and begin to recognize relaxation as giving nothing away (pp. 236–238). Whatever response is chosen to inhibit anxiety, it will need to be thoroughly established (i.e., taught and tested) before proceeding.

Imaginal desensitization. In the standard systematic desensitization intervention, the client first proceeds through the hierarchy imaginally, as described below. Lazarus and colleagues chose to omit the imaginal phase. The inclusion of this procedure is often cost-effective because the *in vivo* desensitization cannot proceed (or proceeds too slowly) without it. However, some people have difficulty creating vivid images and others have difficulty controlling the imagined scenes. There is evidence that Lazarus's client Paul may have been at risk for imaginal school scenes turning nasty.

On the other hand, some children follow imagination instructions very well, and much progress can be achieved without moving out of the office. Briefly, the procedure is as follows. Relaxation is induced in the child. The first item on the hierarchy is described, then verified. The child quietly imagines the scene for about 30 seconds. The next scene is presented in the same way, and so on. Comfort level and relaxation are regularly checked. If at any stage the child feels anxious, relaxation is reinduced and a scene is presented from much lower on the hierarchy before leaving the session. Relaxation should be confirmed and the session end on a note of success. Short sessions twice a week are typical.

Alternatives to the imagination behind closed eyelids include slide shows or videotapes of the scenes from the hierarchy. Clearly these procedures are expensive, to be used in circumstances where the benefits outweigh the costs (e.g., if speed of treatment is critical, or other techniques have failed). In all cases, the objective is to build a history of coping responses with approximations to real-life situations.

Graduated performances. Paul proceeded through the hierarchy as outlined, but gradually, with a large number of intermediate steps. In the first half of the desensitization hierarchy, anxiety was kept at a manageable level by the use of relaxation, the emotive imagery distractions, and the reassuring presence of the therapist. No attempt was made to progress from one step to the next—no matter how small the transition—until the current situation was well established as being under control.

It took 2 to 3 months to establish Paul at school without a chaperone. The anxiety reaction was by and large under control, effectively disinhibiting the social skills he had previously displayed with classmates and teachers. To maintain Paul at school, free of anxiety attacks, the program incorporated contingency management with continued graduated performances. That is, specific rewards were made contingent on school attendance with less and less access to the therapist. After a total of 4½ months (encompassing a number of setbacks) in the program, Paul reached a level of confidence where he agreed that he no longer needed rewards such as tokens and comic books. Ten months later, he was attending school and had made further progress, according to parent report.

Commentary. The above example implies a type or a level of therapeutic expertise not appropriate to some readers of this book. It follows a more clinical, less of a training model than procedures described in other chapters. However, the procedural aspect of graduated performance can be readily implemented by a broad spectrum of childcare professionals. Use of graduated performance does not require highly specialized clinical training, and it is a procedure of considerable power and wide application. All tasks to be learned may be rethought as a series of graduated performances. The basic principle of most value is that any task that causes difficulty can be broken down into subtasks to be trained as a sequence of approximations.

Participant Modeling

Another approach to the treatment of fears, ranking with systematic desensitization in its popularity and proven efficacy, is participant modeling (Bandura, 1986). Briefly, the procedure entails observing someone else's coping skills (usually a peer's), and subsequently attempting to imitate them. Considerable use is made of graduated performances, following a carefully established hierarchy. However, participant modeling is usually classified as a variant of vicarious learning, the principles and practice of which are discussed in some detail in Chapter 3. Clearly the techniques of systematic desensitization and peer modeling have elements in common as well as elements of disparity. A comprehensive approach to treatment is likely to be most successful.

Children Helping Children

A critical variable in determining positive experiences in social interaction is, of course, other people. The anatomy of the social environment of school-age children comprises mostly peers. Thus, collaboration of peers is a powerful way to alter the environment and enhance the experiences of the socially phobic child.

This technique, as developed by Hops et al. (1979), was discussed briefly in Chapter 3. One variation of their procedure was to offer systematic reinforcement (through points or tokens) to peers who successfully encouraged shy children to initiate an interaction. Isolate children will also increase their participation when peers administer reinforcers to them (Smith & Fowler, 1984) or when the peers are rewarded for initiating (e.g., Nordquist & Bradley, 1973). More extensive and systematic training of age-peers to make initiations has proved valuable with severely handicapped children (Strain, Kerr, & Ragland, 1981). A twist to the peer paradigms of particular relevance to the fearful child is the use of *younger* children as playmates. Furman, Rahe, and Hartup (1979) found that organized one-on-one play sessions for social isolates were of greater benefit when playmates were about 1 year younger than the target children. The identification of ideal playmate characteristics deserves more attention, especially for children with severe and specific fears.

The construction of a supportive social environment with peers has demonstrated value in the above cases and in a variety of other social disorders (Strain, 1981). However, this technique is conspicuously underused with children whose social skills are established, but are swamped by anxiety in a narrow set of circumstances. To change the environment systematically would seem to be a treatment of choice. Whereas desensitization introduces the client to systematically changing environments, these environments are identified as they may be found already to exist, not as they may be created. Concentration on building a variably benevolent context may greatly speed up the application of graduated performances. Another approach to speeding up desensitization is explored in the following case study.

CASE STUDY: SCOTT AND THE DOCTOR

Systematic desensitization is an extremely effective but somewhat lengthy procedure. The case cited earlier took 4½ months, with an extensive professional commitment during that time. The general procedure can be greatly abbreviated by incorporating other techniques. The case described here incorporated video recording and a specially selected peer. Thus, its major focus included both graduated performance and the social environment. The results have been previously reported at a conference (Dowrick, 1983a), but are not currently published elsewhere.

The procedure follows the basic desensitization technique, but the imaginal and *in vivo* experiences are replaced with the video medium, and a peer is used to facilitate beginning the hierarchy. The child's attempts to face each level of the hierarchy are videotaped and then edited to show apparent effectiveness at that level. These coping tapes are reviewed by the child several times before proceeding within the hierarchy.

Scott was a 5-year-old boy with congenital physical disorders. He would scream and cry when being taken to medical institutions or when approached by anyone in a white coat or called "doctor." He played very well with his peers, and he would assert himself or cooperate appropriately with other adults. Clearly he had suitable social skills in his repertoire, but completely lost control of exercising them in particular circumstances. Consequently, Scott did not cooperate with the medical profession. His condition was such that frequent examinations were imperative, however, which is why he was referred to me when I was employed at the New Zealand Crippled Children's Society.

Goals

By 6 weeks Scott would visit a doctor or a dentist and show no more apprehension than an average 5-year-old. In 12 months Scott would regularly attend his necessary clinics and cooperate to the extent of allowing essential routine examinations to take place.

Hierarchy

1) Pretend to be a doctor with another child as patient.
2) Play patient with another child as doctor.
3) Allow adult "doctor" to inspect inside of throat.
4) Allow adult "doctor" to put dental instruments in mouth.
5) Visit dentist for inspection of teeth.

Procedure

Treatment of childhood medical and dental fears, as reviewed by Melamed, Robbins, and Graves (1982), typically use systematic desensitization, modeling, or behavioral rehearsal. The procedure developed for Scott provides an unusual combination, through the video medium, of all these approaches. Scott was provided with his own custom-sized white coat and a stethoscope. He was introduced to another child (whose ambition was to become a doctor) who agreed to play patient. Scott was encouraged to role-play the doctor, which he did, with some temerity at first. The exchange was videotaped and edited to maximize his apparent confidence and social skill in the situation. He then reviewed his tape three times during the next week. To edit and review the videotapes was much simpler than the alternative of creating more role plays. It more nearly approximated a coping performance, and the video was considered much more compelling and reliable than scenes from the child's imagination. At the end of the week, Scott reenacted the role-play situation under the scrutiny of independent observers.

He was judged free of anxiety in the reenactment, enabling progress to the next level. (Had he been observed to be anxious, an intermediate step would have been devised.) The procedure was then repeated for steps 2 through 4 on the hierarchy. At step 2, the other child most willingly played doctor, complete with white coat, stethoscope, and band-aids. In steps 3 and 4, a colleague at the Crippled Children's Society (an instructor for the sheltered workshop), whom Scott believed to be a doctor, role-played as required. In each case the videotaping, editing, and review by Scott followed a similar format.

Results

Each week Scott moved readily to a higher level on the hierarchy. Within 6 weeks he visited a dentist, without the dentist's staff being aware that Scott had ever experienced difficulty. Independent observers rated his anxiety as equal to or less than three other randomly chosen children at the same clinic.

His progress was further put to the test spontaneously in the same time period by a need to visit a physician concerning a stomach upset. His mother reported that he coped extremely well, showing apprehension, but able to express himself about it. Overall, Scott's family reviewed his progress in the warmest possible terms, and 12 months later reported him to be expressing himself without fear or tantrums, in line with the 12-month objective.

Discussion

In two other cases, similar procedures have been applied with comparable success (Dowrick, 1983a). One was a 6-year-old girl who had refused dental examinations for over 3 years. The other was a 4-year-old girl who had previously exhibited extreme fears of audiometric testing. Although no control conditions were built into these studies, it seems reasonable to claim that progress was extremely rapid (all were completed within 4 to 6 weeks with only a few hours of therapist involvement) in comparison with reported treatments of similarly well-established childhood fears (O'Leary & Carr, 1982). The use of the peer in the case described also seemed pivotal to the speed of the young client's progress.

CONCLUSION

In some respects, fear of people or institutions can be seen as an extreme case of social withdrawal. Most studies of relevance from the literature on social skills training with children derive from programs for isolate children. However, the established efficacy of treatments for phobias, in which due respect is paid to the specificity of the disorder, provides us with more comprehensive techniques. Social skills training can benefit from the recognition of disinhibition and more use of graduated experiences; conversely, child clinical psychology could benefit from more recognition of social factors and peer help. Altogether, major advantages may be derived from closer attention to the interplay between social survival and phobias – suggesting the emergence of more specialized social skills training programs for fearful children as an area of concern in its own right.

A review of the procedures described in this chapter suggests a *unifying theme*. The graduated experiences of systematic desensitization and participant modeling – with or without peer help – allow *generalization* of a minimal coping response to more demanding situations. That is, repeated experiences in a relatively benign environment strengthen the coping response, making it more robust to variations of context. A new coping ability is thus established, for a slightly more demanding situation. Progress can then be made by strengthening the new coping response and repeating the procedure. This formulation, I suggest, provides an explanatory mechanism for systematic desensitization, at the same time indicating the elements in common with participant modeling that make the two techniques so similar in efficacy.

The issue that remains, then, is not what is desensitization, or what is participant modeling, but what are the superior ways to enhance "experiential generalization." Relaxation, positive imagery, and the presence of a coping model are established possibilities. Variations of medium, such as edited video and the use of peers emerge as further considerations. The techniques reviewed have applicability not only for withdrawn and fearful children, but also when social survival has become limited by aggression.

CHAPTER 5

The Aggressive Child

As with the fearful child, the child who is aggressive is not void of social skills. However, in contrast, the skills are not inhibited but are distorted or misapplied, coming from too narrow a repertoire. Aggression can be seen as a form of social communication that fails to enhance, or even to respect the other party, and that lacks personal control. Children who are aggressive are characterized more than anything by their relative impulsiveness. Many varieties of assessment can be used, behavioral observations being the most popular. The most effective social skills interventions are those that concern control of impulsivity or the intensity of emotional reaction. Impulsivity can be addressed directly by training reflectiveness, or indirectly by training more acceptable reflex actions.

This chapter briefly reviews the most popular ideas concerning the roots of aggression. Methods for assessment, both to screen suitable clientele and to develop intervention procedures, are then described. Interventions most promising for this disorder appear to be those establishing cognitive control. Therefore, some detail is given on self-instruction training, the ability to take another's role, and interpersonal problem solving. The research referred to and the procedures described are most relevant to peer-directed aggression of elementary- and middle-school-age children. (Aggression in the family is dealt with in Chapter 6, and teenage aggression in Chapter 10.)

INTERPERSONAL AGGRESSION

Theories

All theories of human aggression acknowledge both inborn components and the influence of learning. Freud believed aggression to be a fundamental instinct, matched in importance only by the sex drive. He claimed that if instinctive aggression were not released, it would continue to build up in search of an outlet. But even he stressed the role of experience in determining how and to whom that instinct is expressed. The ethologists come closest to a pure instinct theory. The most cited Konrad Lorenz (1966) agrees with the psychoanalysts about a constantly building drive in need of expression. Most ethologists and sociobiologists (e.g., Marler, 1976), however, claim instead a latent tendency that is triggered by specific stimulus patterns. For example, in angelfish male aggression is evident only in the presence of certain displays by another male.

In most species, males are more aggressive than females. In humans this tendency may be due in part to physiological differences (see Kalat, 1984, pp. 312-323). In particular, the male sex hormones (androgens) and low activity of serotonin synapses in the brain (peculiar to males, at least in mice) contribute to aggressiveness. Suggestions have also been made that the male sex chromosome contributes to aggressiveness. This idea originated in the finding that people with XYY chromosomes are overrepresented in prisons (XYY is considered an abnormal configuration – males are normally XY, females XX). However, a closer examination of the facts has revealed that most XYY inmates are convicted of nonviolent crimes (e.g., car theft, larceny), and are of lower than average intelligence. It seems that low intelligence, more likely than "super-maleness," contributes to the incarceration rate.

Moreover, there are obvious environmental factors influencing the greater level of male aggression. For example, male aggression becomes more probable, given that boys are usually stronger, whereas girls are more skilled verbally and are differentially discouraged by society from being physically abusive. There is evidence that girls express more aggression than boys do, through nonphysical means (e.g., social exclusion, Feshbach & Feshbach, 1972). Social learning theory goes further in supporting the claim that aggressive behavior and its alternatives are learned not just during early developmental stages, but at any age; and not just through reinforcement, but through observational learning (Bandura, 1973).

Whatever its origins in the individual, aggression serves a function in the social context. It can be argued that aggression is often a communication – a complex behavior used purposefully to gain benefits for the "communicator." However, it clearly falls short of being a social skill as defined in Chapter 1 on at least two counts. Most conspicuously, aggression denies the rights of the other party and opposes the attainment of mutual goals. Also, the aggressive person often lacks personal control. Aggression, furthermore, leads to social rejection, which may defeat in the longer term some of the aggressor's own goals. Therefore, in contrast to shyness, which manifests as a lack of social interaction, aggressiveness may be best seen as a malfunctioning social skill in need of redevelopment or replacement.

Nature of Aggression

Emphasis on theory in aggression has clarified personal and situational features, but at the expense of attention to the manifestation of aggression as it occurs. A more exact understanding of the aggressive transaction itself will shed, I believe, the most illumination on interventions to change aggressive behavior. Essentially the manifestation comprises a *perceived provocation, emotional arousal, dispersion* of the arousal, and its *consequences*.

Examination of causes or of consequences leads to contradictions. For example, either losing *or* winning in games increases aggression (cited by Bandura, 1973). The notion of catharsis suggests that the witnessing of physical abuse between others will reduce aggressive expression, whereas observational learning theory predicts the opposite. When angry, either "blowing off steam" *or* "counting to 10" can divert aggressiveness, and both response styles are documented to correlate sometimes with increased blood pressure and sometimes with decreased blood pressure. Furthermore, although anger increases the probability of aggression, it can occur with cold calculation.

Social skills training cannot (and ethically should not) be a magic wand that eliminates all vestiges of aggressiveness from a child's repertoire. But it can offer choice. Whereas an increased ability to choose is a major underpinning of all skills-based therapies, the training of clients to recognize an alternative response and its consequences is given special emphasis in working with aggressive disorders. A major reason for this strategy is that aggression often bears the intrinsic reward of success, according to the immediate objectives of the perpetrator.

Choice is appealing when it is recognized that angry or aggressive expression can have negative as well as positive consequences for all parties, particularly in the longer term. For instance, pushing others around can make a person unpopular, thus reducing the chances of cooperation on later occasions. Lack of consideration may occur as a result of poor impulse control (action before thought), lack of alternative responses (inadequate thought), or extreme emotional reaction (disorganized thought).

Some research has attempted to examine these possibilities with a view to their implications for treatment. Peters, Walters, and Bradley (1981) offer an interesting example. They compared 52 socially aggressive boys (8–12 years) with the same number of nonaggressive boys (based on various ratings), otherwise matched for age, grade, and teacher. All were given the following tasks:

Perspective taking: three different tests in the understanding of cognitive and affective cues of others (cf. Piaget's "egocentrism").

Social problem solving: the ability to generate alternative solutions and to imagine alternative consequences to a variety of social situations (cf. Spivack & Shure, 1974).

Impulse control: matching one figure with its mate in a group of similar drawings (MFF; Kagan, 1966); Porteus Mazes (Porteus, 1942); word building from scrambled letters.

No differences were found in perspective taking between the aggressive and nonaggressive groups of boys. The only difference between the groups in their social problem solving was a tendency for the aggressive boys to generate more physically abusive-sounding alternatives as their first listed suggestion. However, there were no distinctions between their most preferred solution nor in the total quantity or variety of solutions. By contrast, differences between groups were evident on *all three impulse control measures*.

The study implies that aggressiveness, at least for boys of that age, is primarily a deficiency in control. These results and others (see review by Urbain & Kendall, 1980) have implications for treatment programs, described later in this chapter.

ASSESSMENT

The major concerns of assessment here are to identify the clientele (who are the aggressive children?) and to identify the issues to be addressed by intervention. In practice, the children are identified all too readily. An aggressive child is not overlooked the way a withdrawn child might be. This step, therefore, is generally not given detailed attention by practitioners. However, there is a range of very useful measures that can be used for this purpose, and they are the methods of choice to evaluate program effectiveness.

Extent of Aggressiveness

The most valuable methods of assessment that provide scores for before-and-after or normative comparisons fall into two general categories: direct observation of ongoing or role-played behavior and paper-and-pencil responses to hypothetical situations by the child or someone who knows the child well.

Direct observation provides the most scientifically valid data, and is recommended as a necessary part of any serious work. Unfortunately, this method is the most expensive and the most difficult for which to obtain reliability verification. Systems of direct observation are usually developed specifically for individual research projects (Van Hasselt et al., 1979). Some are used to investigate precipitating conditions of aggression, for example when children have watched filmed violence (Bandura, Ross, & Ross, 1963). Others examine baseline and treatment effects in natural settings (e.g., Reid & Hendricks, 1973). Childhood aggression has been most extensively studied (through direct observation techniques) in family settings, and therefore more detail on this form of assessment is provided in Chapter 6.

Some attempts have been made to provide standardized procedures for direct observation. Clearly worded checklists of what to look for are supplied, along with instructions of how to structure observation intervals and settings. Those conducted in free social settings (e.g., school recess) have the advantage of a natural setting, but lose on standardization. Clearly, 20 7-year-olds under sunny skies in a two-acre playground offer different possibilities for altercation than 45 teenagers in a small gymnasium after five days of rain. To improve standardization (at some cost to realism), some assessments have been designed for role-play situations. These have the added advantage that they may be videotaped and scored later. The most important advantage of role play over observation in natural settings is that the general range of sample situations (e.g., taunts from other children, praise from the leader of the sports team) is under the control of the data collector.

A good example of a role-play test is the Behavioral Assertiveness Test for Children (BAT-C), developed by Bornstein, Bellack, and Hersen

(1977). Before the test, the procedure is practiced with the child: a scene is briefly described and a "prompt" is given for the child's response. To illustrate, "Imagine you are at the movies, a boy your own age wants to pass in front of your seat and is rude about it. 'Hey, get your feet out of the way!'" The test has been developed to contain 12 positive items (compliments) and 12 negative items (insults, threats, demands). An example from the original (p. 186):

> Narrator: "You're part of a small group in a science class. Your group is trying to come up with an idea for a project to present to the class. You start to give your idea when Amy begins to tell hers also."
> Prompt (Amy): "Hey, listen to my idea."

The child is then expected to respond the way he or she normally would in the given situation. In the experience of myself and my colleagues, we have found it valuable to allow a few minutes of interchange and for the prompt to maintain the role-play character in the interaction. In this way the role-play test provides more information about the child's typical response patterns. This information is valuable for intervention development (see "Planning for Intervention," p. 78).

The BAT-C appears not to have alternate forms, which would provide different role-play situations for before and after evaluations with the same group of children, but it has been chosen frequently for use in studies (e.g., Ollendick & Hersen, 1979). Role-play assessment generally has been criticized for its potential invalidity, in particular, the tendency for subjects to enact (to the extent possible) the response thought to be desired by the experimenters (Kazdin, Esveldt-Dawson, & Matson, 1983). Another evident objection is that role play per se is bound to improve with practice. Since, in the course of training, children usually get a lot of role-play experience, postintervention improvements may not necessarily reflect improved *social* skills. For this reason (and because it facilitates later intervention processes), I advocate training to role play, as a *theatrical* skill, prior to assessments. Possibly the greatest disadvantage of role-play assessment is its time consumption.

Paper-and-pencil tests are even less realistic than are role-play tests, but they have the advantage of easy administration. In particular, a number of children can be assessed through self-report simultaneously, or an informant (e.g., parent, supervisor) can be used. The format is similar to a role-play test in that the child is presented with a series of situations for a response. The major difference for the child is simply that the situation descriptions are read rather than listened to. Another difference is that the child then describes the response, or more likely indicates a choice, instead of reacting directly to the prompt.

The Children's Assertive Behavior Scale (CABS), developed by Michelson and Wood (1982), is a popular self-report measure of this kind. It presents 27 situations with possible responses in a multiple-choice format. For example:

> You know that someone is feeling upset.
> You would usually:
> (a) Say, "You seem upset; can I help?"
> (b) Be with them and not talk about his or her being upset.
> (c) Say, "What's wrong with you?"
> (d) Not say anything and leave them alone.
> (e) Laugh and say, "You're just a big baby!"

The questionnaire may be responded to in two ways: one in which the "someone" is another child and the other as if it were an adult. The forced-choice format limits the range of actions that a child might make, but it does allow for objective scoring. The 27 items are scored on a range of -2 to $+2$ each. The sum of positive values (maximum 54) is the *aggressiveness* score; the sum of the negative values is the *passiveness* score. Responses deemed *assertive* are given zero value. Thus, the test attempts a kind of three-dimensional scaling. (The sample item above is scored: a$=0$; b$=-1$; c$=+1$; d$=-2$; e$=+2$.)

The CABS can also be used for informant reporting. That is, the parent or teacher may provide information about the child through the questionnaire items, given a simple change of wording. In the description of the situation, "you" is replaced by "the youth." In other respects, the instrument is identical. Possible informants also include neighbors, friends, or other people who have sufficient social interaction with the child to be able to make the required judgements. There is reasonable evidence that the data supplied by well-chosen informants is as good as, and sometimes better than, those provided by self-report. However, the word "usually" (present in all items) may lead to inconsistent interpretations and may mask progress between assessments. For example, option (a) in the above sample item may have improved from "never" to "sometimes," but still not "usually."

Planning for Intervention

The above assessment measures of aggression are moderately useful in planning interventions, in addition to their primary purposes of screening and evaluation of intervention impact. To identify a limited number of key social situations that will maximally benefit a specific group of children – and thus clarify the curriculum for a planned training program – a slightly different approach is preferable.

Twenty or more selected situations should be carefully sampled. This number must be reduced to five or ten to be targeted in a training program. In this selection process, it is necessary to examine the individual implications of each situation and the child's reaction to it. The Irish comedian Spike Milligan once said all the characters in his book *Puckoon* could make "good morning" sound like a declaration of war. Likewise, there are many ways of asking "what's wrong with you?" In the course of planning for intervention we must establish how a specific interaction impacts the life of the child: from the child's and from society's point of view.

It is also necessary to recognize that some idiosyncratic reactions are of critical importance for the aggressive child. Typical assessment measures cage descriptions in terms like "someone" and "usually." However, it may be the *specific* person, or the *unusual* reaction that leads to problems. For example, the child may typically react with positive support to somebody who seems upset. But he may be quite intolerant and vituperative with a family member under similar circumstances. And it may be just these situations that lead to the most concern.

A simple way to pinpoint a selection of target areas with greatest salience for a specific group of children is to use the Troubleshooter for the Social Jungle (TSSJ) checklist. Form C (for children 8 to 12 years) of the TSSJ is shown in Table 5.1. The checklist contains 22 items that have been selected to represent the spectrum of situations where impulsiveness or lack of alternative reactions most frequently lead to escalating aggression. Each item is rated twice on a 5-point scale: once for the degree of discomfort experienced by the child in the circumstances, and again for the likelihood that the situation leads to trouble. In addition to the 22 specified items there is an open-ended question to identify troubling situations not covered by the checklist. Very often this item proves highly valuable, by exposing an idiosyncratic concern of the child, but it seems evident that such concerns are expressed only after working through a comprehensive checklist of suggestions.

The TSSJ may be responded to by the child or by an informant. Under some circumstances it is valuable to have both. The child has access to information available to no one else while a concerned adult has a different perspective and a maturity of perception that may add crucial information. Different versions of the checklist have been developed for children of different ages and with different referring problems.

TABLE 5.1
Troubleshooter for the Social Jungle (C)

Here is a list of things that some children find difficult. You will notice that some give you a hard time or lead to trouble, and some don't. That's what we want to find out. We want you to tell us how you feel about each question on the list. If what is described is a bit scary or makes you feel a little uptight or gets you mad, then that's what we call "discomfort." If what is described sometimes gets you into an argument or a fight, or if it gets someone sulky or you get told on, then that's what we call "trouble." So please go over each question and check how much *discomfort* you feel, and how much *trouble* it usually makes. If you have any questions, just ask.

	Discomfort 1 2 3 4 5	Trouble 1 2 3 4 5
1) You want to borrow a toy from someone you don't like.		
2) Your friend wants to take turns with you, using your new puzzle (or bike, book . . .).		
3) Someone visiting your place takes the biggest piece of cake (you are very hungry).		
4) Someone tells you that your picture is the best.		
5) A kid in your class made a super picture, and you feel you should say so.		
6) The captain of a sport team bawls you out when it wasn't your fault.		
7) Your friend's habit of not wiping his (or her) nose is annoying you.		
8) A kid at your school keeps getting in front of you in line.		
9) The most popular girl (or boy) in class teases you about your talk.		
10) Kids in a gang dare you to sneak candy from a store.		

(continued)

TABLE 5.1
(Continued)

	Discomfort 1 2 3 4 5	Trouble 1 2 3 4 5
11) You want to ask a stranger if you can read his (or her) comic book.		
12) You are alone with a cousin and you don't know what to say next.		
13) You don't want to play with your friend because you're still mad at your parents over something.		
14) You're worried about your dog at the vet, when the teacher asks you why you're not doing your math.		
15) Your friend asks you to help with her (or his) homework but you really don't want to.		
16) You are told to wait behind and you really don't understand why.		
17) You wish the person next to you would stop whispering.		
18) A teacher always ruffles your hair and you don't like it.		
19) A child at school has a rough home life and mopes about a lot.		
20) Kids who've been at the school longest get to play in places you don't.		
21) You are put on a team and the rest are all girls/all boys (opposite of you).		
22) You and a friend can go to the movies, but your friend insists on one that you don't like.		

(continued)

TABLE 5.1
(Continued)

23) Are there any other situations that give you a lot of "discomfort" (are scary, or make you mad), or lead to "trouble?" Write one or two here, if you can think of them:

(1) _____

_____

(2) _____

_____

Note concerning the application of TSSJ

The questionnaire is written to maximize the independence of children responding to it. However, guidance and clarification should be offered as necessary. Explanations, examples, and substitutions to wording can and should be made, provided only that the spirit of the questions is retained. For example, most references are to classmates, but the questionnaire could be used in the family setting where it would be more appropriate to sample reactions to siblings, parents, and neighbors. At all times it is valuable to encourage children to offer elaborations like "I don't mind when my friend does it, but when so-and-so . . ."

The intended spirit of each item is as follows: 1) making a difficult request; 2) cooperation; 3) fairness; 4) receiving a compliment; 5) giving a compliment; 6) receiving criticism (unwarranted); 7) criticizing a friend; 8) complaining (not a friend); 9) being teased; 10) peer pressure; 11) politeness; 12) conversation; 13) acknowledging anger; 14) acknowledging worry or sadness; 15) refusal; 16) asking why; 17) changing another's behavior; 18) children's rights; 19) empathy; 20) status; 21) sex differences; 22) conflicts.

The TSSJ Form C is designed to clarify the curriculum of social skills training programs for elementary- and middle-school children who are aggressive or disruptive. It may be adapted for other populations.

In planning a curriculum for a group-training program, all children would complete the checklist and/or have it completed by an informant. An extra copy of the TSSJ can then be used to identify the most significant problem areas, and thus compile a "social jungle curriculum." First consider all open-ended items. Where possible combine them to reduce the number or use them as explications of the more generally worded items on the checklist; give these issues top priority. Next, consider each child in turn. Identify the two or three situations that seem most urgent for that child by combining the ratings of "discomfort" and "trouble" (if in doubt, give priority to "trouble"). Make a frequency count of the most urgent items on the TSSJ Curriculum. Again, items with some similarity or overlap may be combined. The issues that appear most frequently then constitute the curriculum. Finally, the issues should be ranked with the most amenable to change at the top of the list.

INTERVENTIONS

The major ways in which aggressive children can change to their benefit are to become less impulsive and to increase the range of alternative responses to troublesome situations. In addition to the vicarious and experiential techniques described in earlier chapters, an emphasis on recently developed cognitive strategies has proved to be valuable. Cognitive factors allow a child to slow down, to consider alternatives and their implications, thus taking emotional self-control. (Successful and highly documented treatments of aggression have also been based substantially on the restructuring of consequences [e.g., Patterson, 1982]. These are described in Chapter 6 since they have been implemented most frequently in a family context.)

Cognitive Control

In the last 10 years there has been an upsurge of interest in cognitive aspects of human behavior. Child training and therapy strategies have offered no exception. Several strategies of major influence in the treatment of children with aggressive and acting-out disorders have a focus on cognitive control. This burgeoning of interest owes surprisingly little to the field of child development which, under the influence of Piaget, has traditionally given major emphasis to cognition. The impetus has come – even more surprisingly – from a number of behaviorally oriented psychologists, in particular, Bandura, Ellis, Beck, and Meichenbaum. They all claim that attention to thought processes is useful – some say essential – to changing emotions and behavior.

Applied behavioral psychology of the 1950s and 1960s developed along lines faithfully derived from the laboratory (e.g., Lindsley, 1956). The principles of reinforcement, extinction, and environmental control had been fine-tuned on pigeons and rats, without recourse to imputations concerning unobservable cognitive elements. As valuable as these principles have proven (see Chapter 6 for further discussion), by the 1970s behaviorists began to look for more. Two views "legitimized" the incorporation into behavioral science of cognitive processes – previously considered *déclassé*. The first is that thinking may be considered a class of behavior, and thus amenable to behavior change principles. The second is that thoughts mediate behavior, and therefore may be critical to behavior change in some instances.

The champion of radical behaviorism, B. F. Skinner (1953) has described thinking as covert language behavior, and has assured us that "no science of behavior can be complete without an understanding of those processes which take place beneath the skin." By this he did not mean thumping heartbeats or gastric disturbances, he meant cognitions and emotions. If thought is behavior, then it is subject to the laws of behavior change. That is, if specific thought patterns are identified as beneficial to the thinker, they can be helped to occur more frequently with appropriate reinforcement, and likewise deleterious thoughts can be conditioned to occur less frequently. Some behaviorists have pursued this reasoning explicitly (e.g., Wolpe's "thought stopping technique") and others have adopted it implicitly in procedures to be described. Skinner, nonetheless, remains concerned by the current emphasis on cognitions, which he considers to be a bandwagon proceeding in the wrong direction (Skinner, 1983). Wolpe (1983, pp. 114–117) also attacks the philosophical shift to "cognitivism" as a "retrogressive viewpoint." Whatever time tells about cognitive psychology in mainstream behavioral science, it seems to be providing impetus for considerable applied research.

The serious attention to cognition as an essential mediator of action, while articulated some time ago (e.g., Rotter, 1954), has occurred primarily from the influence of Albert Bandura (1969; 1977b; 1986). His position, in contrast to that of Skinner, is that an understanding of the thought processes that link a response to a stimulus is *essential*, rather than incidental, to the science of behavior.

At the same time, another sphere of influence has been felt from theoretical positions even further from the behavioral mainstream. In particular, Aaron Beck (1976) and Albert Ellis (Ellis & Grieger, 1977) have claimed that *all* feelings and actions are the product of cognitions and perceptual interpretations of situations. Their orientation places primary emphasis on cognition rather than the stimulus event. To change behavior, therefore, they claim it is necessary to change thoughts. These procedures, generally referred to as *cognitive behavior therapy*, go further than insight therapy, however. Insight provides information about causes of past behavior; cognitive behavior therapy attempts to change automatic thoughts, which are triggered by stimulus situations, which in turn trigger responses, be they internal feelings or overt behavior. Thus, these therapists propose a paradigm — *stimulus–thought–response* — in which each is automatic or conditioned to the other, with *thought* being the critical link in the chain.

The works of Beck and of Ellis have been most influential in the treatment of adult depression and other disorders. Donald Meichenbaum (1977) has taken their basic ideas, combined them with the theories of Luria (1961), a developmental psychologist, and produced his own distinctive brand of cognitive behavior therapy which has been used extensively with children. One of his major contributions has been the development of a technology used specifically to alter thought patterns that affect impulsivity and emotional control.

Self-instructional Training

The explicit use of cognitive training, or "self-talk," to control impulsivity was first reported by Meichenbaum and Goodman in 1971. The procedure has since been adapted extensively into a variety of self-control programs – including social skills training with children (viz. the "Think Aloud" program of Bash & Camp, 1980, described later in this chapter). The basic procedure of self-instructional training is described below.

The technique is based on two premises, indicated above. One is that action is controlled by conscious or unconscious thought, or "self-instructions." The other is that these thought patterns become automatic (or unconscious) through a process that mimics infant development of self-instruction. As Luria (1961) and others have observed, soon after infants learn to talk they may be heard giving themselves "instructions" – at least they provide a vocal commentary on their own actions, with or without an audience. As children get older, these commentaries become less detailed and less distinct, until they are merely whispered or mouthed before they disappear. It is speculated that the self-talk becomes covert, and finally entirely automatic or unconscious.

The training program, therefore, follows the developmental sequence. First, the trainer models the task and the self-instructions. Motor tasks, such as copying line patterns (studied in the original Meichenbaum and Goodman, 1971 experiment), are most straightforward because the vocalization does not interfere. Next, the child attempts the task while the trainer says the instructions in the first person. These instructions will include directives to slow down, to stay calm, and to correct errors. For example: "This piece is tricky, I will go very carefully and take my time. Now it doesn't matter that I made a mistake, I can just erase it, go over it, and get a nice job at the end." Then the child repeats the task, or similar tasks, several times over while also repeating the self-instructions in the following sequence: trainer and child speak the instructions together; the child says the instructions out loud; the child whispers; the child performs the self-talk covertly.

Because the procedure is learned most easily in application to motor tasks, social skills programs employing self-instructional techniques often begin training with picture drawing or maze solving preliminary to transferring self-talk strategies to interpersonal situations. The skills thus learned facilitate training of the capacity to appreciate another person's point of view and to evaluate alternative responses and their consequences in a given situation. Training to take different roles and to generate alternatives in social situations is discussed before describing the "Think Aloud" program, which combines these two procedures.

It is generally claimed by child development specialists that middle childhood (ages 8 to 10 years) is the time when most children develop the ability to understand other people's perspectives on a situation. This ability is called *role taking*, or sometimes *empathy*. At this age children overcome what Piaget referred to as their *social egocentrism* (Stone & Church, 1984). However, there is great variability in age of acquisition: many children over 10 years old may still impose their own perspective on others, and many children less than 8 will be capable empathizers. In studies of childhood aggression, inability to take another's role has been claimed as a causal explanation of the aggression (Feshbach & Feshbach, 1972).

Elements of role taking are eminently teachable to most children of school age. The ability to understand what someone else thinks or feels is not an all-or-none phenomenon, but has a gradual and variable development. The younger child will begin by appreciating new perspectives most similar to her own. Development will depend partly on cognitive capacity, but also considerably on experience. Training in role taking, therefore, involves providing relevant social experiences and examining them in an educational way.

Programs described in the remainder of this chapter emphasize the use of descriptive scenarios. Through discussion many points of view emerge, particularly in a group setting. *Puppets* are helpful because children attend to them as more clearly distinct from themselves. Social skills training programs for school-age children most frequently include the recognition and expression of emotions in the curriculum. Brief exercises like charades can be devised for portraying and guessing nonverbally expressed emotions. A child's clear and versatile expressiveness is frequently a prerequisite to his ability to recognize the same feeling. Thus, the logical sequence of training is first for the child to practice expressing emotions and motives through the face, the body, and with puppets, then to recognize expressions portrayed by others. Finally, the prediction of thoughts and feelings, given knowledge of a situation and the characters involved, is called for.

Role reversal is another useful training device in the development of empathy. Role playing in which children enact characters other than themselves can be used following or in place of scenarios relevant to the training situation. For example, Freddie may frequently quarrel with a girl at school. After role playing a typical scene, he may reverse roles and play the girl's part while one of the other group members plays Freddie. Discussion of these role plays can enhance empathy, and also provide an impetus for brainstorming, which leads naturally to problem solving.

Interpersonal Problem Solving

Reducing impulsivity in aggressive children will be insufficient in itself if there do not exist alternative responses that these children can evaluate and apply to more socially skilled effect. In many cases, it seems, alternative reactions are already within the skill repertoire of children whose impulsiveness leads them to aggression. But in a significant number of further cases, suitably expressive, but nonoffensive, alternatives need to be taught.

The interpersonal problem-solving training programs developed by Spivack and Shure (1974) (also see Spivack, Platt, & Shure, 1976) provide a major contribution to this purpose. The program uses a script of 17 sequenced games for young children, designed to be implemented by teachers or parents in short daily sessions over several months. Interpersonal problem solving proceeds through four phases: situational analysis; possible antecedents; possible consequences; evaluation. Each phase is accomplished through group brainstorming, and repeated as often as necessary (particularly the last two phases) to reach satisfactory solutions.

Situational analysis. Pictures or games are used to set the scene. Children are asked to describe the scene (e.g., a little girl has fallen off her bicycle) and to suggest what it means to the person (or people) in it. In particular, emotions are identified. (What does she probably feel?)

Possible antecedents. Children are then asked to speculate what might have led to the situation. Physical causes (e.g., a broken bicycle) are called for, and other emotional causes are identified (why else might she feel unhappy?). As with brainstorming generally, the aim of the exercise is to generate numerous possibilities, not to arrive at a "correct" answer.

Possible consequences. The question is asked, what might happen next? Each of these three phases provides practice in thinking about cause and effect, to gain an appreciation that no behavior occurs in a vacuum.

Evaluation. Finally the question is asked, is the suggested action a good idea? Each consequence (e.g., crying, pointing blame, asking questions) is evaluated. Thus the children enlarge their knowledge of and sensitivity to a range of potential responses to different situations.

The general approach of Spivak and colleagues has been to encourage children to reach their own solutions. Where possible, the methods are applied to actual problems faced by children during the training period. The program described below incorporates problem solving with additional emphasis on building skills beyond sensitivity.

The "Think Aloud" Program

A program that explicitly incorporates and expands upon the above cognitive techniques has been developed by Bash and Camp (1980). Earlier studies by Camp (1977) suggested that aggressive children (at least, boys between 6 and 8 years) were as capable verbally as their peers, but failed to use their reasoning ability to control their behavior in provoking situations. The training program (first described by Camp, Blom, Herbert & Van Doorninck, 1977) evolved for use with primary school children in the classroom, but could be adapted for other settings. The program proceeds in two phases that draw, respectively, on self-instruction training, and on social problem-solving.

Self-talk. The first phase addresses a sequence of four questions.

1) What is my problem?
2) How can I do it?
3) Am I using my plan?
4) How did I do?

Training on these questions is first provided for nonsocial tasks, for example, coloring in shapes with a crayon. In this instance, the answer to the first question might be "to color this shape the best we can without going outside the lines" (Bash & Camp, 1980, p. 147).

The second question will have multiple, limited answers. For example, "go slowly near the edge," "hold the crayon so I can see what I'm doing."

During the task the teacher reminds the children (by modeling) to self-instruct. The teacher then prompts question three by demonstrating the response ("I am going slowly near the edge. I can see . . . "), including coping with an error ("Oh no – I slipped over the line. Doesn't matter. I'll watch out").

The final question is evaluated in terms of effort, success, and feelings. "I tried my best. I only once went over the lines. I'm very pleased and proud."

When children are adept at following the teacher, they can work in smaller groups guided by one of their peers as a leader. When they become thoroughly familiar with the self-instruction procedure applied to coloring and mazes, they graduate to social situations.

Interpersonal problems. Social situations are introduced by way of pictures that suggest conflict between children and others in school or family settings. This phase of the intervention follows the Shure and Spivack program with considerable elaboration to the instructional content of the evaluation. That is, the problem situations are analyzed, particularly with respect to the emotional content. Physical causes and emotional antecedents are suggested, and further action and their consequences are speculated upon.

The evaluation of alternative solutions is set against four criteria:

1) Is it safe?
2) Is it fair?
3) How does it make you and others feel?
4) Does it solve the problem?

(In practice, the third criterion breaks down into two: how does it make you feel; how does it make others feel?)

Children at primary school have a good understanding of safety, but may well need additional instruction about fairness. The "Think Aloud" program, therefore, devotes one of its nine interpersonal lessons to this topic. The authors warn that children frequently disagree on what is fair. It seems that the discussion of fairness may be more valuable than reaching an agreement, and the discussion leads neatly into the next criterion. Even if a solution is perceived as fair, it may be recognized as leading to negative feelings for one of the parties involved. Attempts are made to find solutions with which everyone feels happy.

These first three criteria, it would seem, effectively eliminate aggressive solutions. However, some overly passive solutions will likely remain (given that children of this age are relatively unsophisticated on issues of personal rights). The last criterion will question those solutions that keep the peace at the expense of avoiding the issue. For example, if a boy needs to bring his model airplane in from the rain but his mother has just yelled at him not to go outside, quietly saying nothing will not solve the problem.

The cognitive-based strategies described lay some groundwork for reducing impulsivity and expanding the options open to a child facing difficult situations. They also considerably improve the child's understanding of the potential effects that emerge from different social interactions. To achieve adequate behavior change in which less aggressiveness consistently occurs, additional experiential learning must be provided. The "Think Aloud" package, therefore, includes further components, in common with other programs.

Rehearsal and assignments. It is not clear from Bash and Camp's (1980) description how these components are achieved. However, it is clear that the cognitive training strategies can be placed in the general group program model described in Chapter 2 and exemplified in Chapter 3. Role-play situations, taken from the discussion context, can be enacted, providing the opportunity for graduated practice, feedback, and feedforward. Assignments can be made to observe situations of conflict and to report back what happened.

It is obviously undesirable to create conditions of conflict, even for the purposes of peacefully resolving them. The most satisfactory assignments derive from predicting unavoidable sources of conflict likely to occur in the natural environment. For example, a girl may constantly be led into fights with her younger brother who pesters her to play with him – an issue identified during assessment. The circumstances can be brainstormed and role-played within the group session. Specific strategies can then be planned for the girl to try out at home if the relevant circumstances arise. Strategies should be planned that do not overextend the child's capabilities, to maximize the chances of success, to be reported at the next meeting.

These strategies are successful also with aggressive children in older age groups. In particular, anger management developed by Novaco (1975) originally for adults, has been successfully adapted for adolescents (Feindler & Fremouw, 1983). Programs for teenagers are discussed in Chapter 10. Contrasting strategies applied to aggression in the family setting are given some focus in the next chapter.

CHAPTER 6

Children with Adults

In previous chapters social interactions have been discussed most often as child to child. This emphasis has been deliberate. Nonetheless, a highly significant part of a child's life is spent interacting with adults. The type of interaction is qualitatively different, however, and deserves a chapter of its own. The intervention strategies are different, too. Most programs for families are aimed at training the parents directly, and the children only indirectly. As will be seen, most parent training programs, whatever they are called, essentially serve to train communication between the parent and child.

Groups of children with adults may be trained as previously described, incorporating minor adaptations. This chapter focuses on training parents to be more socially skilled with their children.

CHILD-ADULT INTERACTIONS

Interactions between children and adults are essentially different from child-child interactions for a number of reasons. The first is that children have much less power, whereas adults are often in a position of responsibility as well as control. Because of the *imbalance of power*, it is difficult for both parties to be genuinely equally assertive, or socially skilled, as defined in Chapter 1. Parents have power over their chil-

91

dren because of tradition, physical size, age, and economics. As a result, parents can be aggressive ("You do what I say, or else"), or they can over-react to the "unfairness" of their power by subjugating their own rights. Or even worse, they can oscillate between the two. Children, lacking power, may abandon their rights in order to keep the peace, or they may resort to deception or sycophancy to gain their way.

Control by parents would be easy if they wished to have no relation-ship with their children (e.g., build them a small, sound-proof room — which, astoundingly, sometimes occurs). Parent training goes beyond issues of power balance; it is best construed as altering the *quality* of social exchange. In some matters, parents have control, in others, chil-dren have control. What is important is that control is achieved in a mutually enjoyable fashion. To maintain a climate of honest expression and mutual respect requires that parents make an effort and children be afforded constant encouragement. Such a task is difficult, especially as children's needs and capabilities are forever changing with matura-tion. The demands of interaction between children and other adults are similar. Communication with adults who are not parents is helped by a diminished focus on power, but hindered, usually, by less understand-ing.

A related factor concerns the relationship of the child to the adult. In most instances that receive clinical attention, communication break-downs of importance occur in relationships between children and adults in *authority*: family members, schoolteachers, law-enforcement person-nel. These relationships are often ongoing and inescapable. The situa-tion gives rise to an adult perspective that their communication must prevail. What starts out imperative becomes imperious. Communica-tions about setting fires without fireplaces, cheating in examinations, or selling cocaine take on a sense of urgency in which achieving the end may supercede the means. Receiving the message becomes entirely the child's responsibility, and communicating loses its two-way quality. Troubles arise when all exchanges, urgent or otherwise, take on this character.

A final major consideration in child-adult interactions is that they operate *across maturity levels*. There are differences in both the style and the content of language over the life span, most conspicuously in the childhood years. It is not only that grammar and vocabulary de-velop, which is most obvious, but the interests of a person change over time. When I was an 8-year-old, my greatest fascination about choc-olates, which we had rarely, was that *sometimes* they came in foil wrap-pers. I made a collection of all the wrappers I could gather, carefully smoothing out their wrinkles and storing them in a box. This variable focus of interest plays a more fundamental role in communication than is generally realized. The task of the receiver is to perceive and interpret processes that in turn depend upon at least tentatively developed mental constructs. These constructs are the product of a person's interests and previous experiences.

For example, a 4-year-old may not understand such terms as "same" and "different," or "above" and "below" — but not because these are long and difficult words. At 4 years old you can lie on your back on the grass and look down on the sky below. The terms do not have too much importance at that age, a fact easily overlooked, however, in adulthood. Likewise, a teenager, lacking the experience of having total responsibility for another person, will be genuinely noncomprehending of parental concern over unexplained absences. The importance of "at least remember to call if you're going to be late" has to be accepted on faith.

Coercive Families

The majority of cases in which parents take the initiative with their concern for a child's behavior involve complaints of aggression, tantrums, or noncompliance. These parents are usually very willing to become involved in a training program. Often these families follow a pattern of interactions that Gerald Patterson (1976, 1982) and his colleagues at the Oregon Social Learning Center have dubbed "coercive." Coercion means to control by force or threats of pain, and Patterson points to its reciprocal nature in some families.

As mentioned in Chapter 5, aggression in childhood can become a habit because it works. From detailed studies comparing boys referred for treatment with a matched sample of nonreferred boys, Patterson (1976) reported nine behaviors that occurred significantly more frequently among the "problem" boys. Patterson and his colleagues studied a total of 28 behavior categories, 14 coercive and 14 noncoercive. Of the nine differentiating categories, eight were coercive (and interpersonal), such as disapproval, humiliation, noncompliance, and yelling. The noncoercive behavior was self-stimulation. It is interesting to note that the groups in the reported studies could not be differentiated on "appropriate" social activities, such as approval, attending, laughing, and playing. In fact, the problem children complied more often than the other boys, although not at a level of statistical significance.

The basic observation is that problem children communicate very unpleasantly. Others in the social environment then tend to respond by reciprocating the coerciveness. As Patterson puts it: "This process produces extended interchanges in which *both* members of the dyad apply aversive stimuli" (p. 269). Unpleasant interchanges do not follow the patterns of ebb and flow that pleasant exchanges do. It may be quickly found that matched coerciveness most usually ends by one person rapidly escalating the attack. Thus, it is learned that mutually maintained unpleasantness is effectively put to an end by increased aggression.

Overall there is clear evidence that obnoxious child behavior is frequently matched by obnoxious behavior of the parent (or other family members), and that aggressiveness, particularly by older children, may be the result. Under these circumstances, the reciprocal influence may be broken by working with the communication patterns of either party. Sometimes it would be more effective to train the parent, or both the parent and the child together.

Insular Families

Recent research has considerably clarified the circumstances in which parent training is differentially successful. In particular, Robert Wahler (1980) has made an extensive examination of what he terms the *insular family*. By this description he refers to families that have poor social support, citing evidence for unsatisfactory long-term effects of parent training. The sad irony is that it seems the families who most need the help are the least likely to benefit from it. The single parent, lacking financial resources, and whose social exchanges are limited mostly to harassing agencies, stands to gain enormously from improved communication with her or his children. But whereas the skills may be learned in a training program, the probability of implementing those skills in day-to-day functioning is quite low.

Other circumstances have been identified as mitigating against good results. For example, in her review of consumer issues in parent training, Martha Bernal (1984) lists research evidence for the following: marital difficulties, depression, single parenthood, low socioeconomic status, attitudes in conflict with training philosophies, a severely critical view of the child, and unwillingness to devote sufficient effort.

Wahler and Dumas (1984) summarize these circumstances as "multiple coercion." That is, parents may be trained to cope with their child as one source of coerciveness but it becomes exceedingly difficult to maintain their deescalating interactions in the face of coercion from other sources. One approach to alleviating these circumstances is to target a reduction in the additional causes of coercion (e.g., couple counseling, development of social support), prior to parent training. Key strategies in determining how and when to approach these other elements of the behavioral ecology have been investigated in a variety of populations with some promise (see Embry, 1984; Lutzker, 1984).

Another technique to improve parent training, described by Wahler and Dumas (1984), is to help parents to alter the way they characteristically perceive and describe coercive situations by diminishing the global qualities and negative assumptions typically invoked by these parents. For example, a child may be described as "a pest," "always screwing up with playmates," or "thoughtless." These descriptors are too vague to provide the basis for a meaningful intervention, but perhaps more importantly, they promote a mind-set in the parent to draw negative conclusions about the child's thoughts and motives. Wahler and Dumas cite research in which they asked mothers to comment on their children's (seemingly innocent) behavior on videotape. Coerced mothers typically made elaborations such as, "She asked me for something to eat. When that happens, she usually wants me to treat her like a baby. She'll start to whine" (p. 393). These parent observational styles can be systematically retrained. Elements of the above suggestions are incorporated into the section "A Parent Group Intervention" (p. 100).

PARATHERAPY AS SOCIAL SKILLS TRAINING

Parent training – training the parents rather than the children in circumstances described as "child problems" not parent problems – is usually conceptualized as one form of what I term *paratherapy*. That is, the parent is thought to be the change agent, the therapist *in loco*. Other examples of paratherapists are teachers in classrooms or nurses in hospital wards who are trained in a narrowly defined set of psychological principles, because they are in the setting that enables consistent contact. The growing use of paratherapists is a recognition of the fact that effective therapy does not take place in once per week 50-minute sessions. However, whereas this conceptualization is accurate, it may be advantageous to reconsider the concept of paratherapy as social skills training.

Before the 1960s parents were mostly excluded from child therapy. In the following two decades, children tended to be peripheral while the parent received the help. Thus, if parent and child did not get along, either the parent was crazy *or* the child was crazy – the professional attitude was to treat one individual or the other. Most recently, as family systems theory has made an impact (Gurman & Kniskern, 1981; Lutzker, 1980), parent-child problems have become increasingly recognized, and dealt with, as a *social interchange*.

Whether the emphasis is on training significant others as paratherapists or on treating the family as a unit, the child is part of a *system* of mutually influencing components. As important as the components (individuals), are the links between them. The primary element of the linkages that make a family, or larger social unit a system is communication. Thus, for people to operate systemically they must communicate in some manner or another; better communication and, therefore, improved functioning of the system, means better social skills.

ASSESSMENT

The overwhelming majority of research studies in parent training report the use of sophisticated, direct observation in the assessment of parent-child disturbances. However, these studies are essentially of a human laboratory nature in which labor-intensive observation procedures are budgeted for at a cost not to be met in most applied settings.

Karen Budd and colleagues have recently devised an assessment system that promises to be a manageable compromise for obtaining essential data to implement intervention planning, allowing meaningful outcome measurements, at reasonable cost (Budd & Fabry, 1984; Budd, Riner & Brockman, 1983). The system consists of five brief, structured activities, aimed at different potential training strategies. It was developed to suit children 2 to 5 years old (cognitive functioning level). However, it is anticipated that, within the structure of the book, this chapter will be used mostly with families of older children. Therefore, an adaptation of the Budd system, for children of ages 8 to 12 is provided in Appendix D.

Five parent skills are examined:

1) instruction giving
2) differential attention
3) use of contingencies
4) teaching new skills
5) use of time out

These skills are evidently the most important in providing the clarity and consistency of communication by parents necessary for children to feel secure and guided – not coerced – within the family system. As will be seen, they embody many of the microskills identified for adults seeking rapport with children. However, the list is by no means closed. For some populations the ability of parents to play with their children may be a valuable inclusion. But the parent skills assessment as it stands is a most useful *thermometer* of communication areas worthy of attention.

The assessments are best made in the family's home, but may be made elsewhere with the cooperation of parent and child – both of whom should repeat their understanding of the instructions for verification. If an assessment task goes awry, it can simply be started over, following clarification. The observers' tasks are not difficult, but they will require some training, including practice and discussion. Observers need a stop watch and a clipboard with observation sheets prepared for quick scoring on the basis of the lists below. A watch or calculator that can be set to make an unobtrusive tone once per minute is also useful. Each of the five assessment tasks takes between 10 and 20 minutes. Therefore, an hour and a half to two hours should be set aside for the complete assessment procedure.

This assessment tool may be used before and after intervention, and as a curriculum guide to parent training. It will be very evident that it primarily assesses parent deficits, rather than those of the child. Nonetheless, it serves as a guide to improved social skills as a two-way interaction.

INTERVENTIONS

Several distinct approaches are currently in vogue in the training of adult-child communication skills. They include programs based on different theoretical approaches such as transactional analysis, client-centered therapy, and social learning theory. There is value to be found in each of these approaches, of which the social learning, or behavioral, is by far the most thoroughly documented as efficacious, as might be judged from the applied research literature (e.g., see Dangel & Polster, 1984).

As a form of communication training, sound parenting offers *structure*. The fashions of parenting this century have vacillated between the authoritarian and the highly liberal. Recently the strongest advocacy has been to combine the best of both approaches, and the current concensus appears to favor an authoritative, flexible style. Critical to this viewpoint is the distinction between authoritative and authoritarian, and the recognition that children have rights as distinct from children being free to do as they please. Optimally the child will feel secure but be able to exercise control within the structure provided.

The behavioral approach is most well known for its systematic application of rewards and punishments. However, it is useful to recognize that this approach also achieves certain qualities emphasized in communication theory. The use of contingency management provides *consistency* between what parents do and what they say they will do. When families openly discuss the contingencies, it further ensures that parents are consistent with each other over a period of time. Such parental behavior then helps to offer *single messages* rather than double messages to the child (that is, ambiguity between what is said and the tone of voice or facial expression is removed because the contingency agreement makes it clear).

The objectivity of the behavioral approach helps to make explicit what people want of one another and what their likes and dislikes are. It also separates the person from the behavior ("you're lovable but what you did was disgusting"), necessary in addressing antisocial behavior without destroying self-worth. The use of modeling as a training strategy promotes the setting of good *examples*: do what we do, which is also what we say. Furthermore, programs characteristically train family members to structure the expression of negative feelings with *words*: explanations in terms of "when you do that behavior, I feel such-and-such." Conversely, expression of good feelings is promoted *nonverbally* (e.g., smiles, hugs, pleasant activities).

Overall, parent training reshapes the communication patterns between adult and child. One major objective is that the rights of both parties are recognized and facilitated. As a consequence, children should become more expressive and assertive, but accept more give and take and be the source of less friction. In short, parents get to train their children how to get their own way and remain socially acceptable.

Development Patterns

The first part of any parent training program is to assist parents to obtain an accurate set of expectations for their children. A common source of communication difficulties across generations is a misapprehension by the adult of the child's capabilities. An error of overexpectation by a parent is most common in a first child's younger years, or with a child of middle or teen years who shows misleading precocious development (e.g., physical) in isolated areas. Conversely, a child's level of functioning may be underestimated by a parent whose perception of this developing human being grows more slowly than the child does.

Therefore, a brief assessment should first be carried out to ascertain what the *parental expectations* are. This is readily achieved as a by-product of initial interviews and discussions, and during the setting of goals and contingencies. The trainer has a responsibility to help the parent adjust erroneous expectations. If necessary, a brief educational phase concerning social development may be applied. (Table 1.2, p. 12, lists major milestones from birth to the beginning of adolescence. Further details of expected characteristics may be found in textbooks specializing in childhood social development [e.g., Kopp & Krakow, 1982].)

Consequential Training

The vicarious and experiential modes of training have been discussed in previous chapters. The third mode, which ranks with these, is consequential training. It differs from the vicarious mode in that the trainee is active rather than simply observant in the learning process. And it is different from experiential learning in that, as the name "consequential" implies, specific consequences are applied in direct connection with given experiences. That is, when Jeremy asks his sister to choose the television channel during Wednesday evening prime time, he is extended the privilege of watching his favorite cartoon on Saturday morning. This consequence is independent of any intrinsic or incidental reward that might derive from being nice to a sister. The critical factor, therefore, for the trainer (or paratherapist) is not to *predict* an outcome, but to *control* a major part of it.

Parent training, like all good programs, includes all three modes. However, it puts a major emphasis on the consequential mode – the *specific behaviors* that receive *specific consequences* are very openly discussed by all parties concerned. The value of this emphasis is that it provides structure to a situation in which there is an imbalance of power. It may be compared with dealings between big and small nations: If negotiations are public and announced as fair, then the effects of real differences in power are narrowed simply as a function of the process. An incentive structure is established to promote previously disadvantaged enterprises (weak social skills), and systematically withdrawn as these new enterprises become established.

A major strength of consequential training is that its procedures derive directly from the *laboratory*. That is, the application of different types of consequences with different timing, has effects that are well understood, at least by analogy. For example, the pattern of responding during extinction – the rat's frenetic bar pressing, or the child's escalating tantrum – is well known.

However, an unfortunate derivative of laboratory origin is, I believe, the jargon. Even in the most widely used books written and simplified for parents (e.g., Becker, 1971; Patterson, 1975) authors have insisted on teaching the jargon. (A notable exception is a book by Christophersen, 1984.) In face to face training programs, the situation is scarcely different. Bernal (1984) has questioned the value of teaching social learning principles as part of parent training, an issue on which there is minimal and conflicting evidence.

But even when the situation calls for an understanding of underlying principles, there may be more harm than good done by insisting on laboratory jargon, such as "reinforcer," "extinction," "variable interval schedule." The language is polysyllabic and scarcely graceful. Particularly unfortunate is the term "punishment," which in its technical use means simply a consequence that reduces the probability of the behavior recurring. For instance, if a mother smacks a child for teasing his sister, and the boy continues to tease, then the smack is not a punishment but a positive reinforcement. The parent, however, will likely insist that she "tried punishment and it didn't work," for this embodies the usual meaning of the word. Even psychologists specializing in the field confuse the technical term with the popular usage, which connotes obnoxiousness and value judgements. A recent book devoted to the subject and written by notable experts (edited by Axelrod, 1983) is rife with examples.

In the descriptions of parent training programs that follow, some attempts will be made to provide alternatives to jargon.

A Parent Group Intervention

Most training programs have been applied to parents on an individual basis. This is because the majority of reported studies have examined clinical problems where attention to specific issues is appropriate and home intervention is most efficacious. These implementations require a high level of clinical skill and entail a cost commensurate with their urgency.

It is envisaged that most users of this book will be less clinically oriented, better positioned to intervene more at a preventive level, and likely to place a greater emphasis on communication skills per se. Under these circumstances, a group training format is appropriate, although evidence of efficacy is currently quite slight (notable exceptions include Cole & Morrow, 1976; Hall, 1984; Kovitz, 1976). The primary advantages of the group format are the lower cost, the observational learning among parents, and the opportunities for further parent-parent support. Parents sometimes more readily change their attitudes through contact with another parent than with a professional, and parents can be trained to be highly effective leaders of subsequent groups (Raeburn, 1985). However, group organizers will need, for consultation, the backing of personnel resources highly trained in behavioral technology.

The following description is a composite program drawn from clinical experience and from published interventions (e.g., Hall, 1984). It is aimed at parents of children ages 8 to 12, and may be adapted for other circumstances.

Format. The program runs for 10 weeks, with weekly sessions of an hour and a half. The ideal number of participants is eight single parents or five couples. Hall has found satisfactory results with large groups − 25 to 40 participants − but they work in subgroups of five to 12 for most of the session. The format within each session is similar to that for social skills groups for children: review of previous assignments, educational information or scene setting on a predetermined topic, application to individual circumstances, participant efforts at solutions or role plays, feedback, feedforward, setting new assignments.

Preliminaries. The first session is devoted to clarifying parents' expectations of the program, and especially of their children. The first part of the session, therefore, covers the goals of the program and remarks on efficacy of parenting and communication training in general. Then information is provided on the development of boys and girls, of 8 to 12 years old. The experiential part of the workshop is devoted to parental description of expectations and the family-relevant problems. These exercises lead naturally to goal setting as a major task that needs considerable feedback. The weekly assignment for parents is to discuss the goals with their children and to revise the goals using their input.

Clarification. The second session is used to address the issues of behavioral specificity. The primary objective is to train parents to identify behaviors − their own and their children's − with sufficient clarity that all ambiguity is eliminated. This specificity removes much misunderstanding between child and adult: they both need to have identical interpretations of "I get very irritated when you whine." And it lays the groundwork for subsequent objective tracking of patterns of behavior. The week's assignment is to confirm an agreement on goals with further child involvement, and to make a first attempt at monitoring target behaviors.

Monitoring. The next session clarifies the monitoring procedure. It is useful to have one parent bring a child to this session. Drawing on areas of target interest already identified by the group, the trainer can readily arrange role plays with the child in which the parents can practice monitoring for the experience and opportunity for feedback. The week's assignment then concerns more specific behavioral tracking, including antecedents and consequences.

Reacting positively. The fourth session attends to the most important learning principles, but with minimal jargon. The first of these principles is positive reinforcement. That is, some events, made contingent upon an earlier event, increase the likelihood of the earlier event recurring in the future. Saying, "Hey I really liked those friends you brought around this afternoon" may be a positive reinforcer for having home those particular friends. That is true *only* if the likelihood of bringing them back is increased by the remark. For some children, with some parents, the reverse will be true. What is a positive reinforcer is discovered only pragmatically. Thus, parents explore what reactions of theirs are truly positive for their children.

The principles of "grandma's rule" and Premack (1959) are also examined. Grandma's rule is exemplified by, "First you pick up your room, *then* you get to go to the movies." This strategy provides structure and removes the emotional demands of trying to enforce a response on the grounds of a promise, as in, "Okay, you can go to the movies if you pick up your room afterwards." The Premack principle states that any freely and frequently engaged in activity (e.g., watching television) may act as a reinforcer for lower frequency activities (e.g., brushing teeth). Attention to relative frequencies of activities leads to an appreciation of what events are naturally reinforcing, what a child really *likes* to do.

A child may also be included in this session to provide a living example of these principles, and simultaneously to promote opportunities for illustrating the importance of *modeling*, intentional or otherwise. The detail and laboratory jargon of learning theory are neither necessary nor desirable, provided that the trainer has such a crystal clear appreciation of the principles that accurate and convincing examples can be developed relevant to the group members. Parents of children in trouble will have become almost uniformly preoccupied with negative interchanges. This session should serve, above all, to refocus attention on positives in parental behavior and in perception of child behavior. Assignments for the week can be individually tailored to consolidate monitoring skills, with an emphasis on observing and providing positive exchanges.

Charts. The next topic to be covered is that of how to apply artificial incentives for difficult changes of behavior. Strategies of task analysis, which enable large, difficult changes to be broken down into manageable steps, are introduced. Token systems (e.g., points) are explained as a means of reinforcing small elements of progress towards larger goals, which are in turn rewarded tangibly. A primary value of a point system lies in the interpersonal exchange that goes with it, often achieved in some public ritual: for example, a posting of recognized progress on a chart. Therefore the group explores different means of arranging and exhibiting charts to suit the age and personality of their own child. Gold stars on the refrigerator door are not for everyone, but there can be discovered some form of ritual and publicity that enhances the effect of simply keeping track.

Parents frequently raise a concern that offering points and prizes are forms of bribery for what a child should do out of love and duty. Truly, the rewards are deliberately artificial – but then so is monetary reward for going to work. A trainer can say, "Am I being bribed to help you?" A bribe is an incentive to do something *immoral* (or more usually to refrain from what is morally or legally expected, as in bribing an official not to search a suitcase). Points and prizes are merely artificial (usually temporary), but effective ways to *clarify* for a child what is parentally appreciated as signs of love and duty. The weekly assignment is to modify the charting procedure with child input, and to start using it.

Modeling and shaping. The sixth session provides a natural extension of the previous topic. Further exercises are provided on the systematic application of consequences and the analysis and specification of components of change. Opportunities for parents "to set the example," and to teach by demonstration are explored. Parents should be experiencing positive consequences themselves from the improved communication with their children. Much of the session can be spent brainstorming and clarifying specific issues arising from the projects, and individual assignments will derive from these.

Settling conflicts. The topic of punishment, in its technical sense and its common usage, is discussed. This gives rise to two issues dealt with separately. The first is parental *expression of emotion*, particularly irritation and anger. How to achieve this expression, or when and how to control it as a personal right, without damaging the child or the relationship, is practiced in role play. Facilitating appropriate emotional expression in children is then discussed.

The second issue concerns methods of decreasing unacceptable or inappropriate behavior. *Time out*, the most effective and ethical procedure currently understood, is described and demonstrated (a child should be available to take part in this demonstration). Particularly since the children in these families are from an older age group, some of the less well-understood aspects of time out are clarified. Specifically, time out is defined as an environment that is less stimulating or enjoyable than an alternative environment, and the effectiveness of time out depends both on its duration and the contrast between the two environments (Porterfield, Herbert-Jackson, & Risley, 1976). Children go into time out for brief, prespecified periods of time when an established rule is broken. In aggressive families, time out serves to reduce physical abuse by the parent (impulsiveness in all parties is diffused). Thus, the strategy is useful, as much for its effect on the parent as for its effect on the child. Participants in the training group establish the conditions and possible settings for the use of time out in their own families.

Procedures technically called *overcorrection* may also be discussed if relevant to a parent's specific concern (e.g., bed-wetting; Azrin, Sneed, & Foxx, 1974). Overcorrection refers to the restitution of an unwanted behavior's ill effects, plus some extra chore (laundering the wet clothes *and* tidying the room). The weekly assignment is to identify and specify behaviors, if any, that occur with low frequency, but when they do occur, need to be rapidly eliminated (e.g., physically dangerous behavior).

Ignoring. The eighth session concerns more passive means of behavior change. Discussion is provided on the reactions to extinction, and how extinction can occur, intended or not. Extinction (the technical term can be avoided with parents) refers to the disappearance of the "expected" reinforcement for a well-practiced response. Ignoring is the most practical analogue to extinction, but it is important to clarify the circumstances in which ignoring does not make something go away. Ignoring, it must be recognized, is a form of communication. If someone is pulling your hair, shutting your book, and turning up the volume of the stereo, no reaction on your part will be interpreted as some reaction by the antagonist. Therefore, different forms of "ignoring" – quiet responses that disrupt previous patterns of expectation – are planned and rehearsed by participants. Often an acknowledgement helps; for instance, "Look, I know your persistence in the past has gotten you to a movie, but tonight it's 'no,' and I'm going to avoid you until you stop the pestering."

When ignoring is attempted and then abandoned (e.g., trying to ignore whining, before eventually giving in), intermittent reinforcement results. The fact to be pointed out to parents is that this situation (giving in after a delay) actually strengthens the behavior (the whining) and provides very confusing patterns of communication. The assignments are to identify family situations in which this pattern of "failed ignoring" occurs, and to propose solutions to them.

Fading. Programs of behavior change that have been set up with artificial incentives must be systematically altered to fade out the incentives as natural reinforcement takes over. In this session the methods of fading are clarified. Guidance is given to ensure that all parents implement fading strategies, and make specific plans for future revisions to their programs. The assignment is for parents to revise their goals with family collaboration.

Conclusion. The final session is devoted to providing a sense of closure and self-efficacy among the participants. Parents summarize for each other the progress they have made. Each parent is also guided through the process of revising their current goals and establishing future directions. Arrangements are made for continued support and resources for related concerns, with a particular eye for families who may be at continued risk.

Research evaluation data are collected to estimate the impact of the parent training and to revise the content and format for future offerings. Parents suitable to operate as group leaders may be identified. In many ways, parents rather than professionals make ideal leaders. They should be offered training in group facilitation and in the more technical aspects of psychology that are kept deliberately implicit in the program as presented to parents.

Conflict Resolution

Much can be achieved by training parents, in groups, to be better communicators with their children. Naturally, more difficult social interactions will need, or at least greatly benefit from, the presence of the children during training. One procedure that shows promise for its efficacy and economy is conflict resolution training. Suitable clientele are parents and children who show evidence of reasonable communications skills in many circumstances, but who abandon those skills when conflicts of interest arise. Procedures, suitable either for groups of children and their parents or for groups of children only, are outlined below.

Goals. The objective of training is to help families achieve skills that enable conflicts to be resolved, independently of outside intervention, while preserving interpersonal relationships. Satisfactory resolution includes *problem definition, negotiation,* and mutually agreed *action.*

Format. In groups of families (up to four families per group), one parent-child dyad at a time is worked with, while others observe. In children-only groups, various family members can be role-played by other participants. Procedures may be repeated several times to establish skills necessary for independent application by the families in their home settings. Thus, a group can be expected to work thoroughly through the resolution of one conflict with one family, move to another family, and eventually recycle the whole group three or four times, practicing with a variety of example problems. It usually takes one hour to proceed through the first conflict, a process that speeds up fourfold as the trainees become proficient.

Working-together skills. The resolution procedure depends on seven general communication skills to enable working together – skills that must be attended to during training if they are not already in the participants' repertoire.

(a) Be able to own feelings. For example, "I get very angry when . . . "
(b) Talk about others in terms of their actions (not inferred motives or feelings). For example, " . . . when you whistle" (not "you try to irritate me").
(c) Be problem-centered. That is, no sidetracking or blaming while resolving conflicts.
(d) Orient to solutions. Preventing problems in the future is important; the past cannot be changed.
(e) Understand the other person's message. Listen without preconceptions of the issue, and be prepared to paraphrase what the other person says.
(f) Parents: do not patronize. Avoid the use of power to settle a conflict of interest. Help the child to understand the adult view in his or her own terms.
(g) Collaborate. Both parties commit to collaboration.

Conflict resolution practice. The resolution procedure itself takes place in seven steps. These steps are based to a considerable extent on the strategies of problem solving that have proved successful with adult couples (Jacobson & Margolin, 1979).

Steps 1) to 4) define the problem:

1) The child states one problem that gives rise to conflicts. The statement is shaped into the following three parts, with no irrelevancies:
    (i) Begin with a positive remark, relevant to the issue, in appreciation of the parent. For example, "I like how you care about who my friends are." Even "You're a good dad to me" will do, at the beginning of training, with a view to improving relevance later.
    (ii) Express the feeling experienced when conflict begins. Example: "However, I feel ignored and trampled on when. . . . "
    (iii) State the behavior of the parent at the moment of that feeling. Example: " . . . when you say Charley's mom is no good, and then say we won't talk about it."

    The problem statement should be revised until it is completely specific (no irrelevancies), and includes no recriminations. The purpose is for the child to own a feeling and state the circumstances. The parent is required not to say *anything* up to this point.
2) The parent reflects his or her understanding of the child's statement by paraphrasing the original. For example, "You appreciate my concern for the company you keep. But you feel a lack of respect when I mention your girlfriend's mother and want to leave it at that."
3) It may be necessary to have the parent revise the statement of understanding. Common mistakes are to parrot instead of paraphrase, or to add his or her own viewpoint, especially self-justification ("It was tired that night"), dispute ("I said we shouldn't talk about it *now* – that's different"), and countering ("You do the same when we talk about Aunt Lottie"). The child is required to say nothing during steps 2) and 3).
4) The child then either confirms the parent's interpretation or describes what seems to be misunderstood or omitted. In the above example, it may be important to the child that Charley's mother may not merely have been mentioned, but was spoken of disparagingly.

Steps 2) to 4) are repeated until agreement is reached. Only one person is allowed to speak at a time. Steps 5) to 7) negotiate a solution:

5) The parent states a recognition of the situation as problematic to the child. He or she also agrees that since it is a problem for one, it is a problem to be committed for solution by both. For example, "Since this kind of thing bothers you, then I'm prepared to see what we can do differently." The commitment is to work on an agreement that reduces or eliminates *future* occurrences of the type of problem identified. No reference is made to the past.

6) Parent and child brainstorm solutions. They take turns while the parent writes a list. All comments on feasibility and desirability are ignored (and discouraged) at this stage: outrageous suggestions may usefully be encouraged. For instance, the child suggests they hire a butler who will take away Dad's dessert at any mention of closing the discussion. If the suggestions become limited, the trainer and observers can contribute examples. No discussion of the past is allowed, except to produce potential solutions.

7) A solution is agreed upon. First, parts of solutions that are unacceptable to either party are eliminated. Then the remainder are combined, modified, and supplemented to reach an equitable agreement. For example, Leslie will not mention controversial friends at the dinner table; if Dad closes a discussion (e.g., at meals), he will agree to a specific time to continue the discussion later (e.g., Saturday, 10 A.M.); if either party forgets or does not listen, the other gets *all* the Sunday paper until Sunday noontime.

The final change-agreement should:

(i) be very specific, spelled out in clear descriptive terms.
(ii) include each of the following: what behaviors, when they should occur, and how often.
(iii) include reminding strategies – person may not be unwilling but merely forgetful (e.g., agreement may be posted above the fireplace).
(iv) reflect contributions or compromises of both parties.
(v) be recorded in writing, and signed, to increase commitment and reduce later disagreements.

Repetition. The conflict resolution procedure may be slow, hard work to begin with. It is natural that well-established patterns of conflict will be hard to break down. Thus, the new patterns are somewhat mechanically insisted upon in the early stages, but as they become more fluent, they become more fun. All group members take their turn to practice, while others learn vicariously. On the second round, the *parent-child roles are reversed*. That is, the parent's idea of conflict is dealt with. The group situation provides some gentle pressure to be brief and to be fair. In all, considerable team friendship and social support can emerge.

CHAPTER 7

Personal Safety

The term *personal safety* has recently and most frequently come to be used in reference to the avoidance of sexual assault. It is useful in the present context to broaden the reference to include other forms of physical assault by adults. Because of the imbalance of power between children and adults almost the only means of defense for children in these circumstances is some form of social assertiveness. The primary concerns of personal safety to be addressed in this chapter are child abuse, incest, and rape.

There are three quite distinct elements to personal safety training: recognition of the danger; recognition of the personal right to escape; acquisition of specific avoidance or confrontational skills. The assertive skills to be learned vary on the basis of whether the assailant is a stranger or has an existing relationship with the child. In many cases the child has a continuing relationship with his or her assailant.

Situations of incest, by definition, require the child to go on living with the potential abuser or else experience severe disruption in the family. Thus the costs of obvious escape or retaliation are high. Victims of parental physical abuse face a similar dilemma. Children from caring, nonpunitive families can also find themselves victimized, but by people of more transitory importance in their lives: for example, day-care attendants or other adults frequently supervising them. The incidence of rape is almost evenly split between assailants who are strangers and those who are not. Therefore, later in this chapter, there is a brief discussion of elements critical to personal defense against family or acquaintances. The chapter concludes with the description of a specific program for training older children and young adults how to avoid putting themselves at risk with strangers. The program description contains considerable detail which, it is hoped, can be applied to the development of analogous programs for younger children in different settings at risk for physical or sexual abuse.

CHILD ABUSE

According to reports of surveys, in the last 10 years the recognition of child abuse as a "serious national problem" has increased from 10% to 90% of U. S. Americans (cited by Wolfe, 1985). Most likely this finding reflects not an increase in incidence, but a dramatic change in public awareness. Previously (with impetus from the women's movement), rape and spouse abuse had been pulled out of the closet – and perhaps started an important chain reaction of concern about victimization of the more defenseless and vulnerable in society (most recently incest victims and the elderly). Physically abused children currently remain top of the list for public concern.

Incidence

Because so many abuse incidents are kept from public view, meaningful statistics necessarily include estimates as an extrapolation of reported data. The numbers are also necessarily approximate because of differing definitions of what constitutes abuse. The most frequently cited estimate (Straus, Gelles, & Steinmetz, 1980) puts the U.S. incidence at 1.5 million cases per year. In Great Britain, a government report has claimed "nonaccidental injury" to be the fourth leading cause of death in preschoolers (Wolfe, 1985).

The reporting of abuse is undergoing considerable change. A shift in public attitude towards the rights of children (see Chapter 12) – or more exactly, the lack of parental right to treat children as chattels – has hastened legislation mandating reports of suspected abuse. In many states it is now an offense for professionals working with parents or children (e.g., teachers, psychologists, pediatricians) *not* to report to the police cases of suspected physical child abuse. In some respects this legislation will lead to increased exposure of the problem, but it will also discourage abusive parents from seeking help. In some places, court conviction carries mandatory jail sentences. Whatever the true numbers of abuse cases may be, there are too many.

Patterns

Physical abuse occurs in the intersection of three factors:

1) social stress (e.g., isolation, marital problems, financial difficulties, alcohol abuse);
2) aversive child behavior (including misperception of aversiveness through parental overexpectations);
3) parental loss of self-control.

Most cases of abuse involve all three factors in some form, but probably in varying degrees. For example, if factors 1) and 2) increase to an extreme, then a parent who normally has good self-control may succumb to abusiveness. A small but significant percentage of instances result from psychopathology of the parent or extremely harsh, routine discipline. Overall, however, child abusers may be characterized as ordinary people under pressure, on a short fuse, and limited in their child management skills.

In particular, punishment and/or violence is likely to be a familiar part of the lifestyle. All parents necessarily use nonverbal means to manage their children as infants. That is, babies are picked up, moved about, and reoriented physically in the interests of themselves and their environment. If parents do not *socialize* this nonverbal management as the child's language develops, they may use physical punishment, with short-term positive effects, instead. However, the more punishment that children receive, the less responsive they become to it. Thus, physical intensity of control escalates, leading inevitably to abuse. Furthermore, abusive parents were likely to have been abused *or neglected* themselves as children. Whereas the generational cycling of physical abuse has recently been disputed, it is clear that abusive parents characteristically lack a history of empathy and authoritative nurturance in the family.

Treatment

Interventions most likely to be effective are those that target the three factors listed previously as critical to the occurrence of abuse. That is, family and social stressors may be examined first and alleviated where possible. The programs of "Project 12-ways" by John Lutzker

(1984) and colleagues emphasize a comprehensive approach that pays due respect to this factor. Parent training (see Chapter 6) is applied to address the child-manifest problems. This type of intervention is the most cited. Self-control procedures, as described for aggressive children in Chapter 5, are applicable to adults, and form another major component in child abuse treatments. A comprehensive book describing the state of the art is Kelly's *Treating Child-Abusive Families.*

Unfortunately, the treatment of child abuse is very difficult, and the unwillingness of families to participate is disheartening. In some of the most thoroughly researched and carefully implemented programs available (Wolfe, Kaufman, Aragona, & Sandler, 1981), the proportion of referred families who failed to complete their treatment was 87%. Even when families were required by the court to attend treatment, one-third managed not to comply. And naturally, those who comply against their will make poor clients. This bleak situation has been recognized with calls for the urgent study of parent collaboration.

Prevention

In the meantime, vast numbers of children are being abused, many of them chronically, sometimes resulting in severe injury or death. Problems of identification and treatment compliance make it clear that a preventive approach is warranted. Some attempts have been made by child-protection agencies to publicize parent advice- or training-programs that may help parents under pressure before patterns of abuse set in. Social policy has been advocated towards a reduction in all forms of family violence (Gelles, 1982).

I believe an approach with considerable potential is yet to be followed. Children in schools may be taught social skills to minimize the risk of abuse. The major elements would include training to recognize situations of risk, and development of options to deescalate or avoid these situations. These elements are embodied in the training program to avoid sexual exploitation by strangers, described later in this chapter. The curriculum and methods for treating child abuse may be developed by analogy, recognizing that the age group is different, and that dealing with family has special implications beyond those relevant to strangers.

INCEST

The family exploitation problem of incest has even more recently become an issue of heightened public concern.

Incidence

Conservative reports claim that at least 10% of American girls have a sexual experience with a relative, and at least 10% of those have a long-term incestuous relationship with their father or stepfather (cf. Finkelhor, 1979). Other incestuous relationships (e.g., mother-son, brother-sister) occur at much lower rates. Again the available statistics are plagued by secrecy and variable definitions. However, each report that emerges brings forth higher incidence rates (reflecting increased willingness of victims and offenders to admit, at least, to past encounters), which currently stand at 25% for females and 10% for males. Incest does not discriminate against social, economic, or racial groups.

Patterns

Chronic father-daughter incest usually begins a few years prior to the child's adolescence. It typically proceeds from relatively innocent beginnings (additional body contact, fondling). The adult is seldom physically violent towards the child, but is sexually insecure in other relationships (including spouse). He or she is extremely coercive with threats and lies to maintain secrecy.

The child is typically dominated by the perpetrator into secrecy for years; a girl who tries to tell her mother may be (remarkably) admonished by the mother for saying such wicked things about her father. The dependency of the child may go beyond that experienced by victims of other forms of abuse. The adult will claim the sexuality as an expression of love, and the child may genuinely care about him, even if detesting the behavior. These circumstances make it extraordinarily difficult for the child to be assertive. However, some children grow to hate the offender, which at least makes it more possible to break out of the relationship.

Incest victims may be suspected on the basis of changes in social behavior and somatic complaints. As the incestuous relationship intensifies, the girl tends to withdraw, to avoid school, to become especially tense about friendships with boys but show (to others) a precocious knowledge about sexual matters. In adolescence, four out of five runaways, prostitutes, and detained drug abusers are incest victims, according to local agency records, at the time of writing this book. Weisberg (1985), in summarizing the meager available evidence, suggests that 90% of female teenage prostitutes have been victims of sexual abuse, most commonly incest. The incestuous relationship is frequently ended with a pregnancy and a marriage (which allows escape from one abusive household) to a boyfriend who may also be abusive, as the young woman carries with her guilt, low self-esteem, and difficulties with all forms of intimacy.

All states in the United States require reporting of suspected incest. Many have mandatory prison sentences for offenders, and courts may require immediate physical separation of the family members upon allegation.

Treatment

Most usually, treatment begins on an individual basis, then may proceed in groups—all victims; all offenders—and eventually culminate with family therapy. The success rates claimed in terms of lack of offender recidivism are remarkably good, as high as 98% (see studies cited in Mrazek, 1983). However, the punishment for relapse or recidivism is so severe that one wonders if the legislation makes the most critical contribution to therapy. Little research has been published on the success or otherwise of treatment for the victim. Whatever the rate of success or its contributing factors, treatment is provided to the small percentage of incidents brought to judicial attention and to almost no others (since it is illegal not to report suspected offenses). Thus, thousands of cases a year go undetected, or recognized so late that most of the psychological damage has been done.

Prevention

Ultimately, the only means of substantially reducing the incidence of incest, as with physical abuse, is *prevention*. Again, some beginnings have been made with educational programs in schools. These are primarily consciousness raising in their focus. Dolls, comic strips, and plays may be used to illustrate the difference between affectionate and exploitative touching. Some emphasis is put on children's rights of objection to being touched in ways that they find unpleasant, and a strong sense of permission for them to object, or to report instances of exploitation, is conveyed.

Clearly, such education has the beginnings of a specialized assertion training program. The explicit or implied elements of recognizing risk, the personal right to object, and taking action to stay safe are the same elements featured in the program description later in this chapter. I strongly advocate, however, that programs be much more intensive and thorough than the majority of those now offered. Aside from a strong sense of distrust in human relationships, the most severe psychological repercussion of incest is guilt. The risk of partial training in avoiding sexual exploitation of any kind is that, along with the sense that "I could do something to prevent it," comes the feeling "I *should* do something to prevent it." I believe there is some danger in consciousness raising that is not followed by adequate skills training. This danger can be averted by programs that ensure that a skills criterion—rather than a knowledge criterion—is reached by all participants.

Given the remarkable patterns of transmission of abusive behavior from one generation to another, it seems that to develop the means to break those patterns would be one of the most valuable contributions that psychology could currently make to the world.

FAMILY AND "FRIENDS"

When a child is taken advantage of or treated carelessly or brutally, two obstacles emerge that interfere with a child's natural defenses. First, the perception and understanding of the situation is considerably confused. Adults, particularly parents, are necessary to children as protectors and providers. It may be irreconcilably difficult for a child to discover that adults can also be self-serving—at the child's expense. Second, any reaction that the child has to the abuse has implications for other facets of the child's life. Often in cases of incest, the parent and child will have a pact of secrecy. The child knows, explicitly or by implication, that disclosure of the secret may result in other forms of abuse and the loss of some of the protection and provision upon which she or he is dependent. For example, sometimes a father will tell his daughter never to breathe a word to her mother because "the shock would kill her."

Treatment and prevention programs, therefore, must first heighten children's sensitivity to exploitation or neglect without destroying their basic sense of trust. That is, the child must learn that family and friends may offer much that is truly supportive—house, education, recreation—but sometimes behave selfishly through abuse or neglect. Although the selfish behavior is reprehensible and must be diminished or stopped, the support may be valued as positive qualities that most adults offer most children most of the time. Or even though some adults behave so badly that society will punish them with a prison sentence, there are other adults who may be trusted to care.

Furthermore, the training needs to provide the skills necessary for a delicate maneuver. The child needs to be able to avoid the abuse, perhaps to report it to (another) family member, without putting herself or himself at further risk in the relationship. It is generally impossible for a 9-year-old girl, for example, to have the perspective to decide whether or not she is better off with an abusive parent or in a series of foster homes for the next 8 years. The assertiveness necessary for a child to express herself or himself in these circumstances may very well be misunderstood because of the power imbalance. Thus a specialized and difficult social skill is called for when children are at risk in their own homes. Procedures may be adapted with care from the following program.

STAYING SAFE WITH STRANGERS

Following is a description of an intervention program and an indication of its results. The program was developed in Anchorage, Alaska in 1984 for a young adult developmentally disabled population. The inherent difficulties of training this population make the described program necessarily detailed. Therefore, it can be easily adapted with simplification for use with other groups. The project was based on an established sex education curriculum (Newton-Alrick, 1982), enhanced by videotaped feedforward (see Chapter 11).

Rape

Anchorage Police Department statistics for 1982 show that the incidence of forcible rape in Anchorage was the highest in the nation. On a per capita basis four times as many sexual assaults occurred there as in New York City. The official statistics for sexual assault are made far worse by the fact that many rapes are not reported to authorities. Estimates on the proportion of assaults that actually come to the attention of the criminal justice system range from 10% to 50%. Therefore, the reported incidence of 158 rapes in Anchorage in 1982 suggests that the actual occurrence per annum is between 300 and 1,500, as well as can be estimated.

Disability

No information is available from police records about how many disabled people are represented by the above figures. However, based on national statistics, the incidence is likely to be proportionally greater for the developmentally disabled among the population (see Stuart & Stuart, 1981). This subpopulation is less aware of insincerity in personal interactions and less equipped to resist exploitation when they are aware of it. With increasing emphasis on deinstitutionalization for developmentally disabled people, more of this population are receiving independent living support but are less closely protected in the community. Along with greater opportunities for employment, education, and recreation, older children and adults with disabilities are increasingly exposed to danger from many sources.

Sexuality

Sexual abuse of developmentally disabled persons has long been recognized by professionals as a chronic problem. However, the problem has been compounded by myths and lack of information. Relevant information is frequently withheld by caretakers or parents based on erroneous assumptions that the disabled person has no real sexual drive. It is often assumed that a disabled person would be confused by information about sexuality, or that he or she would become sexually promiscuous if given more information.

Intervention Program

The training was provided by the Image Center, in collaboration with the University of Alaska at Anchorage (Dowrick, McManus, Germaine, & Flarity-White, 1985). A videotape, "The Elements of Personal Safety Training," illustrating the critical components of the program, is available.

Trainees. Nearly thirty teenagers and young adults were drawn from the clientele of Hope Cottages, a nonprofit corporation caring for the developmentally disabled. The clients, two-thirds of whom were female, were aged 15 years and over. Some lived in group homes, requiring considerable personal supervision. Others were living independently in apartments, and employed in selected, supervised positions. All were considered by Hope Cottages personnel to be "at risk" for sexual exploitation.

Procedure outline. The clients were trained in six small groups, three to seven people in each group. Six to eight trainees per group would be manageable, but we ran a number of smaller groups to enable better refinement of procedures and to train Hope Cottages personnel in all aspects of the program. Groups met only once for two or three hours of training. In this session trainees were taught to recognize the sanctity of her or his own body and that they had total personal right to its control. They were then guided through role-play situations in which they were accosted by a stranger. The role plays were videotaped, enabling self-model films to be made for feedforward purposes. The self-model videotapes were systematically made available for review by the clients as their final phase of training.

All trainees were evaluated with a series of standardized role plays before and after training. Progress of selected clients was more intensely examined under multiple baseline conditions and with probes in the clients' environment.

Self-values. The session begins didactically, to teach or reaffirm the major concepts of self, safety, and the right to refuse. The group is led, ideally, by male and female coleaders, who can demonstrate issues as they arise. The criteria for the *concept of self* are that the clients recognize how personal their own body parts are, that they can describe aspects of their person that they like, and that it is *their* responsibility to give (or not to give) permission to others to touch them physically. The concept of safety is then explored in a discussion of safe versus unsafe behavior and the probable consequences of each. For example, staying on the sidewalk is safer than walking in the street, reducing the likelihood of being hit by a motor vehicle. Examples of unsafe behavior include getting into a stranger's car.

Finally, the concept of the right to refuse and resist personal demands is explored through discussion with illustrative "threats" from the group leaders. For example, "I'm going to cut all your hair off, okay?" Examples are shifted from the very obvious or aggressive to the more subtle and coercive. The criteria for the discussion of *personal rights* include demonstrations by the trainees that they can say no assertively and that they recognize the right to say no in situations that put them at risk.

Role plays. Discussion is then mixed with role plays, during which the action is videotaped in preparation for self-modeling. Role plays include a male training assistant, whose only interaction with the trainees is to play the "stranger." Various scenes are set and carefully explained, such as going to a bus stop and waiting for a bus. The stranger may then approach the young person and make friendly conversation. The stranger may suggest that since the bus is late, he can offer a ride in his car. The trainee is given considerable flexibility in deciding how to respond at different choice points in the interaction. However, whenever the client acts on a choice, a group leader asks, "Are you safe?"

The role plays, using props, are varied by setting different scenes such as going to work or using a public telephone. The encounters are varied further by altering the tactics of the stranger; for example, he pretends to have lost something on the ground and asks for help in searching for it. Finally, the encounters are escalated to the point of physically grabbing the client. All clients should demonstrate a variety of refusal reactions: loud verbal responses, pulling away, screaming, and running. The clients are trained to show some ability to choose and to act assertively on that choice, the level of proficiency depending on the person involved and the time available. For these purposes it serves to have the most capable trainees practice first to provide models for the others. It is not necessary, however, for clients to reach criterion in all possible situations (which would take hours with that number of low functioning trainees). In fact, it can serve quite well to have some behaviors enacted in isolation, as indicated below.

Feedforward. Role plays are recorded on video for the purpose of creating self-model tapes. The objective of such tapes is to show the trainee responding to risky situations with choices that are appropriate for that client. The responses, based on safe choices, should then seem both effective and credible.

With fairly effective trainees, this objective will be readily achieved using intact role plays. In other cases it will be necessary to edit the tapes extensively. For feedforward purposes, as explained in detail in Chapter 11, it is of no consequence that component behaviors as seen on tape may have occurred in role play in a different sequence. As an extreme example, a convincing shout of "no, keep away from me!" may have been elicited by the sudden appearance of a furry tarantula (obscured from the camera) or simply by a prompt from a trainer, later edited to appear as the response to the stranger's attempt to take the trainee by the hand. Nor does it matter if many of the responses were elicited by demonstrations or prompts, deleted from the self-model tape. What does matter is that the recording represents a credible sample of *future* adaptive behavior of the trainee (hence, the term *feedforward*).

The edited tapes are between 2 and 3 minutes long. The trainees review these tapes at least once every two days for two or three weeks. In some cases, trainees were lent copies to use on their home video machines, requiring but a telephone call to the house parents or the clients themselves to remind them to play the tapes. In other cases, an assistant met with the client to show the video recordings.

Evaluation. All trainees completed the program and met their goals for progress as determined by Hope Cottages personnel. Some showed remarkable gains with a high degree of generalization to the environment. (Manuals and videotapes are being prepared as an instructional package.)

The trainees were assessed before and after intervention as follows. Eight standard role-play scenes were described, in turn, to the client. For example, "This man is a stranger. This piece of carpet here is like the sidewalk, and here is a newspaper. You are going down the sidewalk to get a newspaper. The stranger comes up to you . . . just act as you normally would do. Have you got that?" Each scene was checked out before enactment of the role play (e.g., "Who is this man?"). The stranger was role-played by an assistant not used in any other part of the project. The role plays included a range of requests, demands, and physical coercion by the stranger. The same scenes were provided before training began and after the completion of the feedforward phase. The role-play director emphasized authenticity, not safety, being careful not to endorse actions as either appropriate or inappropriate.

Video recordings were made of these standard role plays. The before and after recordings were scrambled, and the tapes were rated by independent judges. Ratings were made on the basis of specific behaviors that did or did not occur (e.g., saying no loudly; getting into the stranger's car), leading to safe or unsafe conditions.

Under the standard role-play evaluation, 90% of the trainees improved. The remainder rated safe in all role plays at pretest and at posttest, our criteria not being sensitive enough to track the progress of the more advanced clients.

To gain a better understanding of the relative contributions to training from the different phases, multiple baseline assessments were made with some trainees. (For a detailed report see Dowrick, McManus, Germaine, & Flarity-White, 1985.) In essence, the multiple baseline allowed us to compare the gains made from group intervention (instruction and role play) relative to those made from feedforward training. The same role plays were used as in pre/post assessments. It is clear that in most cases the greatest amount of learning took place through self-modeling: for some trainees the responsiveness to self-modeling was strikingly evident (we now need to seek the characteristics of this subgroup).

With some trainees we hope to set up social validity probes. That is, adult male assistants (university students unknown to the clients) would offer rides in their motor vehicles to the clients who were waiting in public places. These encounters would be videotaped unobtrusively.

Some social validation has become spontaneously available. In one case a Hope Cottages client not in the project was sexually assaulted. It was reported that her friends who were in our program found their self-model tapes and reviewed them. They then telephoned the assault victim to console her and to make reference to adaptive reactions as depicted on their videotapes. Cases of client-initiated review of self-model tapes constituted an unexpected but welcome subsequent effect of the program, as did the use of the tapes as a point of reference.

In another case, a trainee "graduate" of our program asserted herself against harassment by a man in a grocery store, eventually going to the management when he would not leave her alone. She was described by Hope Cottages personnel as being generally unassertive and of low self-esteem a year earlier. Her descriptions to her house parent of what happened at the grocery store focused on the self-model as a reference for adaptive behavior.

CONCLUSIONS

Social survival training appears to have a promising place in the prevention of abuse and harassment. Whereas the incidence of such offenses may not be rising, the reporting of them certainly is. The occurrence of physical abuse within families and sexual abuse from any source is now recognized to be of far greater proportions than ever previously countenanced. When these events are known to take place within the family, a remedial approach that addresses both children and parents is clearly to be advocated (see Chapter 6 for major elements that might form the basis of such an approach). In cases of uncooperative parents, interventions must deal directly with the children to develop their capacity for taking care of themselves. When the potential for abuse resides outside the family, or to afford a measure of prevention against the beginnings of abuse inside or outside the family, direct intervention with children themselves is the only recourse.

CHAPTER 8

Disturbed Children

The majority of emotional disturbances and some medical disorders have implications for social adequacy. Regardless of whether a child's level of interpersonal functioning was originally the cause or subsequently the consequence of the disorder, social factors often contribute to maintaining the disorder and interfere with therapy.

Childhood disturbances are by no means necessarily the product of inadequate social skills. Such disorders may require any of numerous available psychological or medical treatments. However, in some instances, social skills training may be the intervention of choice; in many instances, attention to the interpersonal environment may be critically important as an adjunct to therapy. The purpose of this chapter is to identify disorders (not described earlier in the book) that may be recognized as childhood disturbances and that may be significantly helped by attention to social skills. Some guidelines are provided on assessing the likelihood that attention to social functioning will be of value. Finally, methods are described that are most beneficial in the identified circumstances, with particular attention to procedures that build self-esteem.

TYPES OF DISORDERS

A wide variety of childhood disorders have been helped by the application of social skills training as part of treatment. It is convenient to divide those to be discussed in this chapter into three categories, on the basis of whether the deficits infringe on others or self, or whether the disturbance represents unusual psychopathology.

Disorders Affecting Others

Disturbances to be discussed in this section include hyperactivity, impulsivity, attention deficits, learning disabilities, and dishonesty. Delinquency in teenagers is not discussed here but is a major topic of Chapter 10. These conditions are disturbing to the children who manifest them, which should be the main reason for deciding to intervene. However, the most usual reason for referral is that the conditions are made worse by the impact they have on others. That is, social relationships are disrupted, the child is perceived as a nuisance to others, and finally a concern emerges for what the child is experiencing. It is common, then, for the child to receive unpleasant social reactions that worsen the child's original disturbance. Several studies (e.g., Green, Beck, Forehand, & Vosk, 1980) have found that children with outwardly directed disturbances are even less popular with their peers than children with inwardly turned problems, such as shyness.

Attention disorders. Hyperactivity, impulsivity, and attention deficit disorder all have much in common. The controversies surrounding the terminology (see Barkley, 1981) are not important here. Of more importance is the *characterization of social interactions* found in children given these diagnoses by the childcare profession. A noteworthy aside is that boys comprise 80% of these diagnoses, and boys are less socially skilled on average than girls in the same age group.

Children with these diagnostic labels tend to be disruptive because of their activity level, and they appear inconsiderate by their impatience and forgetfulness. They are frequently treated with medications (see Chapter 12), or contingency-management programs (cf. Chapter 6). These treatments, when applied carefully to individual, properly diagnosed cases, are generally quite successful (see reviews by Barkley, 1983; Ross, 1981). However, satisfactory effects take months, sometimes years to accrue, and although some aspects of the problem become more manageable, they never disappear (Douglas, 1980). In the meantime, the targets of conventional treatments are usually confined to the excessive activity level or the deficits in attention, not the skills of social interaction.

The foremost difficulty experienced by overactive and impulsive children in social interaction is the propensity to escalate aggressive encounters. Fortunately, these children are a minority. Most preschool or early school-age children respond to demanding interactions (aggression or snatching by peers) with deescalation. Studies (reviewed by Campbell & Cluss, 1982) indicate that 80% to 90% of potentially provoking encounters lead to a nonphysical response or sometimes rough-and-tumble play. In contrast, children who tend to act physically and impulsively are more at risk to end up fighting. The likelihood of a nonphysical reaction to an aggressive demand is much lower. Moreover, if their demands on other children are responded to by rough-and-tumble play, the likelihood of play being misunderstood and turned into hostility is much higher.

An obvious approach to the escalation problem is to reduce impulsivity per se. Methods for this purpose are described in Chapter 5, in particular *self-instruction training* (Meichenbaum, 1977) and *interpersonal problem solving* (Spivack & Shure, 1974). Self-instruction training has focused on the content of what people say to themselves in a difficult situation. But, irrespective of its content, the self-instruction takes a moment to occur, particularly in the early stages of training. Thus, impulsivity is affected. There are a few studies that claim that the content of self-talk is irrelevant to its usefulness in reducing escalation, that it works simply by slowing down the situation.

Interpersonal problem solving trains children to recognize more aspects of the situation and to generate more alternative solutions. In addition to the direct benefits of both these skills, reaction time is again slowed down. It takes time to consider the situation more thoroughly, and the decision time before reacting increases by the square of the number of alternative solutions generated.

Other factors that may become a consideration after the impulsiveness has been reduced include the ability *to perceive the situation* accurately (discussed in the section "Psychopathological Disorders," p. 130) as well as the *range of alternative responses* in the repertoire. Whereas treatment of these factors is obvious for children referred for social aggression, it may be overlooked for the child labeled *hyperactive*. The importance of these factors is stressed here, not just because the hyperactive child is socially disadvantaged, but because these factors interact with impulsivity. Time spent assessing the situation and evaluating alternatives cannot be spent in physical reaction.

Another approach to attention-disorder deficits is suggested by the studies of Walter Mischel on *self-control* in children. His conceptualization of what is generally referred to as self-control is the ability *to delay immediate gratification* in favor of a larger but more distant reward. He has not used clinically identified populations, but he has systematically studied factors that alter children's ability to delay gratification.

For example, he has investigated the effects of what a child thinks about while waiting for alternative rewards. If pictures of the "grand prize" are made available, children will generally be able to delay longer. However, if the children in these circumstances are prompted to think about the desirability of the prize (e.g., how sweetly marshmallows melt in the mouth) the delays deteriorate (Mischel & Moore, 1980). The findings of these investigations suggest that delay of gratification may be a response class that can be trained. This response class would seem to have obvious importance for impulsive children, particularly in social contexts.

A method of training self-control apparently overlooked in the treatment of attention disorders is to create an audience for the child. That is, there is good evidence that children learn self-control in some situations if they expect to report on their actions later (Risley, 1977). This process is called *correspondence training* (correspondence between saying and doing), described in Chapter 9. Indeed Karlan and Rusch (1982) have made a strong case for correspondence training in such problems as "controlling aggressive, off-task, or bizarre" behavior (p. 161).

Learning disorders. Children are classified as having a "learning disability" not because of low intelligence, but because of *inconsistencies* in the acquisition of academic skills – language and mathematics, in particular. It is not to be confused with an overall developmental delay, as applies to mental retardation (see Chapter 9). These children have much in common with those discussed in the previous section. Therefore, some of the aforementioned strategies may be useful, at least to the extent to which activity level and attention deficits apply to the learning-disabled child in a specific instance. However, one factor likely to be of more importance to the child with peculiar inconsistencies of learning ability is a potential deficit in being able *to take someone else's role*. Given that learning disabilities derive from perceptual, information processing, or retrieval dysfunctions, it is likely that misjudgements of another's point of view will arise.

There is at least some experimental evidence for this logical premise. Dickstein and Warren (1980) claim that learning-disabled children lag behind the role-taking ability of their age-mates. Dickstein and Warren were able, therefore, to compare two groups of children, one with learning disabilities, one without, in which all children were of "average IQ." In testing children ages 5 through 10 years, they found 8-year-olds with learning disabilities to function as normal 5-year-olds. Furthermore, role-taking ability did not seem to improve after age 8.

Training children to perceive a situation from another's viewpoint by taking the other person's role is described in Chapter 5. There is no predicted impact on the academic component of learning disability for this training. However, the impact on social appropriateness and its ramifications for general functioning of the child may make the training crucial.

Dishonesty. Stealing, lying, and cheating can be difficult disorders to treat in young children. For example, John Reid and his colleagues found that procedures (discussed in Chapter 6) of proven value for childhood aggression in the family could be adapted with difficulty and modest outcome to children who steal (see Patterson, 1982). Patterson notes that the majority of parents whose children become chronic stealers do not see stealing as a problem, whereas parents of aggressive children are much more likely to be concerned. To get treatment compliance of the child under these circumstances may be particularly difficult, and, naturally, interventions have little success when they are imposed to preserve social order, and not with the wish of the client.

However, the difficulties faced by traditional treatments emphasize the value in identifying social interaction deficits as a major target for intervention. There is some evidence that very young children (6-year-olds) can easily distinguish between moral rules and conventions, and that they do so on the basis of recognized affect. Arsenio (1983) has claimed that children associate negative affect with a moral rule (e.g., stealing is bad), while a neutrally affective state establishes a simple convention (e.g., riding on one side of the street is pragmatic). These findings suggest that for children whose socialization is sufficiently developed for them to be easily inhibited from moral transgression, dishonesty may still occur if affective states are poorly recognized. The inability *to recognize one's own or another's emotional state* is common in more psychopathological disorders, and is therefore discussed in more detail in a later section of this chapter.

Dishonesty also occurs amongst some children who are perfectly well aware of the moral sanction. It may be that in their perception crime does pay and it is then very difficult for the child-care agent to arrange superior incentives and payoffs for honesty. One approach is for a therapist to review the development of prosocial behavior (see Staub, 1980).

A more profitable strategy may be to train cooperation as a response class, perhaps through games. Unfortunately, most parlor games for children (or adults) are competitive and can be won only at the expense of another player's loss. The proliferation of these games leads to a distorted view of the world. Exceptions, such as the Prisoner's Dilemma, illustrate that we can often gain more by cooperation than competition. That is, by helping someone else a person gains more than by taking something from them. Such a situation is more characteristic of life than the typical parlor game, particularly in families, schools, and jobs where we tend to have repeated transactions with the same people. In writing this book and sharing my thoughts and experiences with other child-care agents, I gain far more than by trying to keep secrets to myself for some "competitive edge."

Patterson (1982) has observed a continuum of behavioral development that might be labeled a *dishonesty dimension*, and that is distinguished from other social disorders. He notes that lying and stealing occur most frequently with children who sooner or later commit vandalism. His data indicate that in about 80% of the cases, children with problems of theft previously were considered problematic for lying and for breaking windows. And a like percentage of firesetters were previously accused of stealing. Thus, violence against objects, rather than humans, is on a dishonesty continuum, not an aggression continuum, a finding that has implications for early intervention.

Very possibly the best strategy with a child who has acted dishonestly is to examine the goals of that activity. Perhaps to lie, steal, or cheat was the simplest way to achieve those goals. A broader repertoire of social skills may expand the possibilities of goal attainment without the risk of moral sanction. For example, if a child cannot ask a parent for money, then he will likely steal it. If a child lacks the social skills to apologize for breaking grandma's vase, she will blame the cat. A social skills training approach to dishonesty is probably one of the most promising and least explored interventions to contemplate.

Disorders Primarily Affecting the Child

The conditions of childhood described in the preceding section are most frequently brought to professional attention because of their impact on the environment. Help is also sought for conditions that primarily affect the child with less impact on others. Many of these disorders have medical origins or consequences.

Weight disorders — obesity and anorexia nervosa — and stress-related medical disorders, such as asthma and diabetes mellitus, have important social interaction components. As the booming field of behavioral medicine (alternatively called health psychology, etc.; see Russo & Varni, 1982) reminds us, psychological factors frequently are responsible for emerging behavioral patterns that subsequently are responsible for health – or loss of health. For example, anger is a noted stressor responsible for the onset of asthma attacks (Melamed & Johnson, 1981) – although, surprisingly, social skills training per se has provided virtually no application in the treatment of childhood asthma (cf. review by Creer, Renne, & Chai, 1982).

The primary contributor to these psychological factors is quality of social interaction. Not only may social ineptitude contribute to behavior undermining a child's health, social difficulties can frequently be a consequence of medical disorders.

Weight. A child not popular at school may seek comfort in extra calories from the refrigerator. Mom probably offers food as a source of love. Or a child frightened by the family responsibilities of growing up too soon may starve herself to gain control or delay maturity. Social difficulties, particularly in the teenage years when peer acceptance becomes especially important, are obviously a source of stress, and therefore a contributor to stress-related disorders.

No programs that I can find have reported on the use of social skills training for children with weight disorders. However, the potential clearly exists. In the family systems approach to treating anorexia nervosa (Minuchin, 1974), the major focus is to change interactional patterns between the client and significant people in her or his life.

Diabetes. In the behavioral treatment of diabetes, more attention is currently being paid to the reduction of stress from improved social interactions. In the United States, 100,000 children and adolescents suffer from diabetes, for which there is no cure. Diabetes may be controlled, however, by adjusting the blood sugar level through insulin injections, diet, and activity. As children grow older, the need for self-management of diabetes control increases. By about 9 years of age, children also need to develop peer relationships in which there is acceptance of the disorder.

Alan Gross and his colleagues have produced some interesting studies on the training of social skills with diabetic children. As a rationale for their work, they cite studies (e.g., Swift, Seidman, & Stein, 1967) that correlate interpersonal problems with poor diabetic control. Although it may seem obvious that medically disordered children who also have social deficits should benefit from skills training programmed around social aspects of the disorder, such interventions have been rarely reported.

In perhaps the first published social skills training program with diabetic children, Gross, Johnson, Wildman, and Mullett (1981) worked with five insulin-dependent children, aged 9 to 12 years. These children – three girls, two boys – were selected because they were suspected by their pediatricians to experience social embarrassment over their disease. These suspicions were verified through parental report and from a role-played assessment. Eight role plays were used in a format similar to the Behavioral Assertiveness Test (Bornstein et al., 1977; described in Chapter 2), but with direct relevance to the management of diabetes. For example:

> You feel an insulin reaction coming on in class. The teacher sees you starting to eat a piece of candy. She looks at you and says,
> Prompt: "What makes you so special to be able to eat in class."

> You are at a friend's birthday party. When the cake is served, one of your buddies says,
> Prompt: "Come on, you have to have some cake."

In this type of assessment, the interviewer describes the situation as set out in the narrative, and an assistant speaks the prompt to draw a role-played response from the child. Gross et al. used eight such scenarios as before and after measures in their intervention. Each role play was rated on eye contact, duration of speech, and "appropriateness of verbalization."

Five of the scenes were chosen at random for intervention. Training, mostly through modeling and role play, took place in a group format over 5 weeks, with two 45-minute sessions per week. What appear to be clinically valuable improvements were made in all scenes, including those three that were not trained. Following intervention, the parents were asked to practice the scenes with their children – an assignment perhaps even better to be given during training. An interesting follow-up validation was made after another 5 weeks, by taking the children to Wendy's hamburger restaurant for a celebration meal. It was contrived that each child ordered unobserved by the others, and the restaurant manager (collaborating with the experimenters) pressing each in turn to buy a milkshake. All children refused the manager's urgings (the children were, of course, later given explanations and hearty congratulations for what had taken place).

Thus, children can demonstrably be trained to be more skilled in social factors surrounding the management of their disease. The obvious next step is to investigate the impact of this training on diabetic control, which Gross and colleagues have begun. Unfortunately, they have so far failed to measure significant improvements in hemoglobin levels of children trained by their methods (Gross, Heimann, Shapiro, & Schultz, 1983). A possible reason for this finding, pointed out by the authors, is that their hemoglobin measure reflects level of blood sugar averaged over time – a function of overall diabetic management – whereas the social skills training addressed only the most stressful threats to diet control. That is, the overall poor disease management of these children overwhelmed the impact of the interpersonal training. It certainly seems warranted to investigate the diabetic response to interpersonal functioning in much more detail. In the meantime, we may be grateful that a beginning has been made.

Psychopathological Disorders

The two-way interrelationship between psychopathological disturbance and social skills has been given more attention by researchers and writers than the disorders discussed earlier in this chapter. Study of the area has consolidated in the last two decades with systematic investigations of adults (see Liberman, Neuchterlein, & Wallace, 1982), and attention has increasingly turned towards childhood conditions over the last few years. In many cases the studies refer to "emotional disturbance" or "psychiatric disorder" without elaboration. The treatment of the topic here will be confined to psychotic precursors, with brief reference to depression, selective mutism, and gender identification. I assume that these disorders disturb social interactions and make them erratic, rather than provide fundamental impediments to the acquisition of basic skills. It seems useful here to make a categorical distinction between childhood disorders that distort the use of social skills and those that delay skills acquisition. Autism, for example, clearly belongs in the latter category, the implications and applications for which are described in Chapter 9.

Our understanding of adult disorders makes very clear the role of social interactions. Poor social exchange often maintains the disorder, prevents therapeutic progress, or induces relapse after therapy. Thus social skills training may be essential to treatment. Furthermore, some of these serious disorders are an advanced development of less serious problems, such as anxiety or withdrawal, described earlier in this book. Or the emotional disturbance may be directly caused by serious problems of interpersonal (particularly family) communication. In either case, the early identification of disturbances and social skills training with children may have important preventive value.

This conceptualization provides the theme for this section. That is, each category of disturbance is examined for the basis of its development from milder disorders and the causal or maintaining role of communication problems, with implications for treatment.

Psychotic precursors. Serious disorders of relevance here include various forms of schizophrenia, passive-aggression, obsessive or compulsive behavior, hysteria, and agoraphobia. Although some of these classifications would not be termed "psychotic," they are extreme disorders, requiring intensive, individualized treatment. All have antisocial elements of either mistrust or coerciveness in which the client may be seen as either victim or protagonist.

A substantial body of work with adults by Vaughn and Leff (1976) and others has drawn attention to the role of interfamilial communication in maintaining schizophrenia. What has been termed *expressed emotion* is one of the best predictors of relapse for discharged schizophrenics. This concept refers to the content and nonverbal components of communication by relatives towards these clients. These findings have added impetus to programs aimed specifically at training social skills in adults with schizophrenic disorders (e.g., Liberman, et al., 1982). Social skills training may be the major form of treatment or it may supplement drug therapy and other interventions.

The proven success of social skills training with these adults supports the possibility that communication disorders may have a role in the development of schizophrenic behavior patterns. Although theories subscribing to a physiological basis for schizophrenia are most commonly supported, one quite popular theory posits that the disorder is a psychological one deriving from specific communication harassments during childhood. The harassment is termed the *double bind* (Bateson, Jackson, Haley, & Weakland, 1956), in which both parents are usually guilty. The term implies that a communication demanding a unitary response is sent such that a double communication is received, and, furthermore, the components of the double message conflict with each other, making it impossible not to offend. For example, "do not read this sentence" is an often quoted double bind. More commonly in a family context, a mother might say, "Yes, you can take the car" in a tone of voice that implies the son should not have asked. The teenager can then catch the bus and offend his mother for not accepting her generosity, or he can take the car and feel guilty in the recognition that she resents it.

When a child cannot physically escape constantly double-binding communications, so the argument goes, schizophrenic withdrawal provides a release. For example, the message that a child is unwanted suggests the necessity to leave the family — but desertion would be seen as the ultimate insult to parental love and sacrifice. It becomes impossible to leave and impossible to stay. One's own world, away from reality, seems very attractive, and the episodes of bizarre behavior that go with it may (ironically) draw more caring and support than otherwise received. The argument is appealing, if unproven. Whether or not these conditions are sufficient or necessary for schizophrenia to develop, it is clear that such communication styles are evident in many families and would indeed exacerbate any tendency to psychotic withdrawal.

In a review of the links between schizophrenic symptoms and family interaction patterns, Falloon, Boyd, and McGill (1982) identified the following features as most noteworthy:

1) discord between parents;
2) overprotective, intrusive mothers;
3) deficiencies in parents' communication skills;
4) poor problem solving abilities.
(p. 121)

The program they have developed is, therefore, family-based. It has five major components, two concerning the understanding and medical control of schizophrenia, one dealing with crises, and two dealing with social skills: communication training and problem solving. Their early results seem very promising indeed, especially with respect to relapse prevention. However, their clientele includes only families in which the dependent offspring are at least 18 years of age.

It should be evident that the earlier the training of social skills is available, the better. Parents can be taught to clarify their communication, in particular to avoid sending one message with the verbal content in conflict with another simultaneous nonverbal message. And children can be taught to seek clarification and to express their own thoughts and feelings when they experience the double bind. This straightforward and logically advisable approach has been conspicuously overlooked in this context.

Social skills training has been used, however, for other psychopathic precursors, with both adults and children. Hersen (1979) has claimed that the "level of premorbid social competence in a hospitalized psychiatric patient is the best predictor of his posthospital adjustment" (p.

189), regardless of diagnostic label or type of treatment during hospitalization. He based his conclusions on an extensive review of published case studies and experimental research. The reports include mostly successful social skills training approaches to such disorders as depression, alcohol and drug addiction, personality disorders, and explosive anger, as well as schizophrenia. None of the work reported was done with children. Rinn and Markle's (1979) chapter, published in the same volume as Hersen's, reviewed the research with children and found it "sparse but promising" (p. 127) at that time. They reported no use of social skills training for children with psychiatric disorders, but a few studies have gone to press since the review.

More recently, Monti, Corriveau, and Curran (1982) described their program for training adult psychiatric patients in social skills. Their basic structure for a 10-week group program with instruction, modeling, role play, feedback, and homework assignments, is similar to that generally advocated in this book (see Chapter 2 for an outline of components). They list 10 topics for 10 sessions. These are:

1) starting conversations
2) nonverbal behavior
3) giving and receiving compliments
4) negative thoughts and self-statements
5) giving criticism
6) receiving criticism
7) listening skills and "feeling talk"
8) being assertive in business situations
9) close relationships
10) intimate relationships

My own preference is to develop a curriculum around the individual needs of group members. But the list is illuminating because it was developed and modified on the basis of a series of carefully evaluated training programs contrasted with other training methods (e.g., bibliotherapy) and control groups. Thus, it reflects the issues typically of benefit to this population. It is interesting to note that the curriculum holds no surprises compared with those developed for other populations.

In general, Monti and colleagues were able to demonstrate clearly the effectiveness of the program, in its impact on social skills of psychiatric patients, and on the general status of their disorders. The program was developed for adults, but the studies did include some clients in their late teens and many with very few years of education. Clearly the program could be adapted for use with a younger age group. Issues raised by topic 8 (business) could be redeveloped for the school environment, and the method of approach could naturally be adapted along the lines of those used with other children.

A comparison may be made with a program described by Jackson (1983) for adolescent psychiatric outpatients. This group program runs about 16 weeks in a youth club setting, with a curriculum built around the participants. Jackson offers very clear details of procedures, which are largely coherent with those recommended elsewhere. An interesting addition to her program is the club setting, which allows extra time with the youths for informal activities including games (e.g., charades; a card game called "Killawink") that are chosen for the enhancement of social skills. The case studies she describes are of "psychiatric disorders" milder than those discussed earlier in this chapter. Elder, Edelstein, and Narick (1979) describe case studies of four adolescent psychiatric patients. These teenagers were long-stay hospital residents, of unstated diagnosis but histories of aggression, and were successfully treated individually with standard social skills training procedures.

A few studies have reported direct intervention with different aspects of social functioning in preadolescents with emotional disturbances. Burnett (1978), for example, found small group training of interpersonal skills to be effective as measured by improvements in speech latency, speech disturbances, frequency of requests, and assertiveness. Small (1979) found both social skills training and interpersonal problem solving to be effective, at least with respect to the number of alternatives that could be generated in given situations.

A promising area for social skills intervention is *childhood depression*. The interrelationship between social deficits and depression in adulthood has received much attention, spurred by Lewinsohn's (1974) persuasive use of social activities as a primary mode of treatment. In a review of social skills training for psychiatric patients, Brady (1984) points out other treatment approaches to depression, such as cognitive therapy (Beck, 1976), including substantial social skills training components. Some programs, with promising results, have specifically targeted interpersonal functioning of depressives (e.g., Hersen, Bellack, & Himmelhoch, 1980; Sanchez, Lewinsohn, & Larson, 1980), but I find none with children. However, at least one assessment study has suggested the value of social skills training for depressed children. Helsel and Matson (1984) assessed several hundred children to evaluate a "child depression inventory." A subset of these children (ages 4 to 10 years) were also evaluated for their social skills. Childhood depression, they found, correlated positively with impulsiveness but negatively with "appropriate social skills."

Another area in which a social skills approach may be taken is *selective mutism* (also called elective mutism). This disorder is one in which children demonstrate good communication skills, but only in certain environments. For example, a child may talk freely at home but be mute at school; another may speak with family but remain silent among peers. These cases are distinguished from social withdrawal by the contrast in speech production and the specificity of the mute-inducing environments.

Despite the obviousness that this disorder exemplifies the failure to generalize adequate interpersonal functioning, social skills training remains virtually untried. Psychotherapy, contingency management, and wait-and-see seem to be the most common approaches, but to which the condition does not readily respond (see reviews by Kolvin & Fundudis, 1981; Kratochwill, 1981; Labbe & Williamson, 1984). A study of two children in which selective mutism as a problem of generalization across environments is treated using self-modeling (Dowrick & Hood, 1978) is briefly described in Chapter 11.

Finally, *gender identification* deserves some consideration. Variously called *inappropriate gender behavior*, and *cross gender identification*, the problems manifest by some children adopting extreme mannerisms, usually stereotypical rather than typical, of the opposite sex, are thorny ones. Concern has been raised and strongly debated for the ethics of intervention (Nordyke, Baer, Etzel, & LeBlanc, 1977; Rekers, 1977; Winkler, 1977). I believe the approach with greatest validity and utility is to consider cases individually on the basis of social deficits (cf. Ross, 1981). Problems of ethics and the best interests of the child can be comfortably addressed by focusing on social skills and expanding the repertoire of choices available to the child in a broad social environment. A case study in which a 4-year-old boy is taught how to be entertaining to himself and others without reliance on girl-stereotyped toys and clothing is described elsewhere (Dowrick, 1983c).

An interesting angle that may be of particular value in working with disturbed children in general comes from the suggestion that their *abilities to recognize emotions* are less accurate than those of other children. Zabel (1978) reached this conclusion following a study of elementary and junior high school children. He used photographs widely employed in studies of the recognition of basic emotions (Ekman, Friesen, & Ellsworth, 1972). Recognition of sadness, fear, and disgust were significantly poorer amongst children previously identified as "emotionally disturbed" in comparison to other children. At about the same time, Morse (1976) reported training 8- and 9-year-old, emotionally disturbed boys to discriminate and label feelings. Appropriately selective feedback was found to be effective for this purpose, but the effects on pathology are unclear. Strategies for training empathy (for which the recognition of emotions is prerequisite), are described in Chapter 5.

In summary, the value of social skills training with a variety of psychopathologies and their precursors probably has much more potential than thus far realized. Reasonably systematic data exist for adults but not for children. However, the evidence from effective programs for adults with, and children without, severe disturbances, converges in support of existing programs that have been adapted, with little modification, for children with developing psychopathology. The most urgent avenue of program development is the systematic study of adaptations to improve effectiveness. There is some evidence that the recognition and expression of emotions in self and others is a valuable place to start.

ASSESSMENT

It is not appropriate to the scope of this chapter to offer tools adequate to the proper assessment of emotional disturbance. But it may be valuable for readers to develop an appreciation of when social skills training is likely to be a suitable adjunct to other treatment. It will be obvious that social skills training should be considered when there are social interaction deficits. However, it may be less obvious that social exchange deficits should *always* receive the benefit of social skills training. That is, even when these deficits are primarily the result of some other disorder, they will not disappear with the removal of the cause. For example, if a magic pill were to cure hyperactivity, obesity, or schizophrenia, the communication deficits born of those disorders would remain in need of direct attention. Thus, the final confirmation of the need for such treatment will be a regular social skills assessment as described elsewhere, with modifications to its administration as necessary.

Major indicators that should draw attention to the possible necessity for thorough social skills assessment include: inability to take a role, inaccurate perception of emotion, and low self-esteem. These issues are identified elsewhere in this chapter in the context of intervention. Below is a checklist of considerations.

Before considering social skills in this context:

• screen for medical factors
• if IQ less than 80, see Chapter 9

Consider social skills training if child has:

• poor self-concept
• poor judgement of mood or attitude of others
• inappropriate reactions to social situations
• inability to take a role
• poor ability for interpersonal problem solving
• excessive susceptibility to peer pressure
• strong outward or inward reactions to rejection
• high frequency of self-deprecatory statements

When these conditions apply refer to an assessment procedure to quantify the impressions.

SELF-ESTEEM

A number of specific procedures are of particular value in the development of programs for children with severe psychological or medical disorders that disrupt social functioning – although I speculate on these procedures in the face of very little data. Procedures that directly address role taking, problem solving, and the judgement of social situations are described in Chapter 5. A further issue of apparent special consequence to children in the present context is that of self-esteem. Because self-esteem may be related to social skills, both as a cause and as a consequence, it is valuable here to summarize some of the procedures used to develop a positive self-image in children. The discussion is applicable to any child with poor self-esteem, regardless of the presence or absence of other disorders.

Causes of Low Self-esteem

In general, low self-esteem is experienced by children as a result of certain kinds of rejection and their interpretation of those rejections. The damaging kinds of rejection are those that result in loss of membership to a group, reflect lack of competence, or lower the worth of the individual. The interpretation depends on the value ascribed by the individual to what is lost or by whom the rejection is expressed. Loss of self-esteem is inevitable if the group is prized, the behavior seen to lack competence is highly valued, or the personal devaluation comes from someone the child looks up to. (See Felker, 1974 for an extended discussion with a similar viewpoint.)

Low self-esteem tends to be self-perpetuating. That is, in a child with a low self-opinion, new experiences tend to be interpreted in ways that confirm that opinion. When the low self-esteem (LSE) child is criticized, whether it be for failure at mathematics or for having too many freckles, he or she is likely to ascribe the basis of the criticism to constitutional factors – to personality traits that suggest personal culpability. By contrast, when offered praise the LSE child is likely to attribute external causes. The high score in the math exam was luck and Aunt Cecilia said my hair looked pretty because she's so sweet and generous. As Zimbardo (1977) has pointed out, under these circumstances, honest, positive feedback has little impact because even complimentary evaluations will be misattributed. The LSE child is searching for acceptance based on an ideal. Since the ideal is built from a combination of the best attributes of many heroes, it is never attainable; thus, acceptance is not a possibility. And so down spirals self-esteem to lower and lower depths.

Solutions for Heightened Self-esteem

From its self-perpetuating nature, LSE can be usefully conceptualized as the *condition*, or state, of the child. This concept provides a basis for understanding the causal and maintaining factors. However, it is even better to think of LSE as a *process*, when considering interventions and solutions. In a sense, the child is "LSEing" the environment.

There are five basic goals to reversing this process. These are set out below, each with two exercises so that one self-esteem exercise may be included in each session of a 10-week program. At all times it pays to be "Rogerian" – that is, empathetic, accepting, and attentively listening. For the programmatic development of high self-esteem it is useful to take a cognitive-behavioral approach. That is, progress must be planned to proceed in small steps, with ample reinforcement for more adaptive ways of thinking and behaving.

Goal 1: Distinguish "Self" From Action

It is typical to confuse the value of one's actions with personal worth. To help reverse the LSE process it is essential to hammer home a distinction. The child must learn that committing a stupid *action* does not make her or him a bad (or even stupid) *person*. First, the difference must be pointed out to the child. Second, helping adults should make a practice of reaffirming the child's worth at the same time as referring to behavior that may need to be changed. For example: "Taking Wendy's jumping bean wasn't fair, but even if what you did was wrong, you're still a valuable person, and we care about you." Finally, the child must be helped to make those distinctions even when others do not. Our lives are full of people who will say "You are a rotten prune" (or worse), when we do something objectionable. To preserve our self-esteem we must learn to take the insults to our person and reascribe them to our actions.

A related trap, as mentioned earlier, is to assume personal responsibility for errors that really have an external cause. Children can be helped to become more realistic in this respect. If a child trips and spills the milk, it is not because she is a clumsy dolt (personality trait). It may be because she did not look where she was going (behavior). Or it may be because she had too much to carry and the rug was out of place (external cause). Some children gain a positive attitude from being put on medications, for instance, for hyperactivity, simply because it relieves their sense of guilt. They have been given a cause for their clumsiness that does not reflect on their morality. To improve self-esteem the cause of embarrassment or criticism should be realistically ascribed to behavior or to external factors, never to personality.

Exercise 1. Find the positive.

Every effort is praiseworthy, regardless of the outcome. In the social skills group, identify some task attempted by one of the members. Choose an event that all participants know about, or one that can be described (it need not be a social interaction). Have the group brainstorm the virtues of the effort. Draw out praise by asking the following questions. What do you like about the motivation for the effort? What do you like about the plan (the objective)? What was the best aspect of how it began (a friendly smile, a clean sheet of paper)? The best aspects of how it proceeded? Of how it finished? What was most positive about what the child felt afterwards?

After brainstorming one event from the past, make an assignment for the future. Have each child take down the list of questions. The homework for the next session can then be for each individual to apply these questions to a task of their own.

Exercise 2. Discard lousy labels.

Choose one of the children in the group with higher self-esteem to start. Ask him to label himself (e.g., I am dreamy, I am clumsy). Get him to explain why he uses that label by giving examples. Then ask him to discard the label and replace it with behavioral descriptions: what he does/thinks/feels in which circumstances. For example, I start thinking about what's on television when the teacher explains the math problems. Or, I feel embarrassed when I knock the paints over while I'm setting up for art.

When one child has a good idea of how to replace a label, ask him to help another person in the group to do the same. Proceed until all children have had a turn. For homework, the group members all may write down examples drawn from labels put on them by other people between sessions.

Goal 2: Distinguish Own From Others' Values

Our accomplishments and possessions have virtues that we must recognize, without being bound by the values of other people. LSE's should first recognize that success is relative and personal. For someone who could only dog-paddle last season, to swim one length of the pool is a marvelous success. Children can also discuss "less than 100% is okay." Even our greatest heroes fail sometimes, and they are not good at everything. The final legacy of allowing ourselves to be dominated by the values of others is that we feel guilty. Children can explore the difference between feeling sorry for having caused another person harm and feeling guilty simply because someone else disagrees with them.

Exercise 3. Set your *own* goals.

Help a selected child to set a goal, and truly explore whether it is according to the individual's values. For example, a child may want to join the hockey team. Force a contrast with the felt priorities imposed by others. Perhaps his father was a high-school hockey hero; perhaps the boy would rather be a computer hack.

Exercise 4. People don't have to agree.

Draw an example of an issue about whose worth two group members have different opinions. Establish that both children are right. It may be useful to compare issues or goals about which adults disagree. For example, owning a sports car or a station wagon both have their virtues, as does living in the country or living in the city.

Goal 3: Breed Success and a Sense of Progress

Progress is *felt* only when accomplishment is recognizable. Therefore, children must be helped to set reasonable goals and to break them down into small, manageable steps. Again, it is essential to emphasize the positive. As any progress is made, children can be helped to recognize success as the product of their own efforts, not of luck. No matter how small and manageable the step, success will not always occur. Make failure positive: it gives data to revise one's plans. Focus on small subgoals that provide a high rate of success.

Exercise 5. Make and take compliments.

Have the children work in pairs, taking turns. One child says something nice of the other and the second child responds without self-effacing. Build a list of 10 compliments each. Then each child can choose a short list for himself or herself of the five compliments they like the best.

Exercise 6. Imaginal self-modeling.

A group leader can demonstrate by describing a recent situation, and improving the outcome with a suggested alternative. Ask all children, in turn, to identify an event that did not work out perfectly for them. Get the group to brainstorm potential, more desirable outcomes (after the excitement, guide readjustments to the solutions in proportions realistic for each child).

Have children close their eyes and imagine it all. Check out the imagery and ensure its success. As a homework exercise, children can spend some time each day with their imaginal self-modeling scenes, gradually enhancing them to keep ahead of their progress in the real world.

Goal 4: Develop a Sense of Control and a Sense of Belonging

A sense of helplessness may result from excessively worrying about the past. One approach to overcoming this problem is to have children identify a source of defeat and have them take the other person's role. The present also causes frustration when goals never seem to be achieved. These defeats usually create a distancing from schoolmates, and even from family. But a sense of defeat comes from having the wrong goals or viewing them inappropriately.

Exercise 7. Process not outcome.

Previously set short-term goals can be reexamined in terms of what will be attempted and how much time will be spent, not in terms of what will be accomplished. Spend time with each child on this exercise. Their homework can be to bring back examples.

Exercise 8. Sharing success stories.

Each child in the group identifies a success they had in the last week, and tells it to the group. It does not matter how small an event it was. If a child has difficulty, encourage the group to help out. Repeat the exercise several times: use as an introduction and reintroduce it on other days. Vary each round with a different theme or time frame: for example, yesterday, on vacation, before Christmas.

Goal 5: Be Your Own Best Friend

Pair off children and have them recall Exercise 5 on compliments. Have each make compliments of the other, and the other write them down. Then each child should add one more positive self-label. Ask each child what time he or she takes for himself or herself. What do they do with that time? Ask them if they ever give compliments to themselves. Compare the power of Muhammed Ali: "I am the greatest!" Everybody is great some of the time.

Exercise 9. Half-empty is half-full.

Identify some events that the children see as failures. Point out that all failures are partial failures. Therefore, any failure is a partial success. For example, 5 times wrong out of 10, means 5 times right; even 10 wrong out of 10 means that you attempted something very difficult. Seek examples and contributions from all group members. The homework can be to bring back more examples and to practice positive self-talk associated with these events.

Exercise 10. Failure is never typical.

Help the children to identify dozens of "easy" successes, taken for granted; for example, getting to school, playing a game. When failures crop up in the discussion, point out that these are the minority, but it is easy to focus on them. We need not be blind to failures, but they should be kept in proportion. Have children complete sentences that confirm their strengths. For instance: Something I can do now is. . . . I could teach or help someone to. . . . Nobody can make me. . . . I feel best when. . . . For homework, practice self-talk for success and self-talk for failure.

Conclusion

Positive self-esteem essentially derives from positive experiences, not from explanations. The explanations simply serve to motivate the experiences. Success in gaining control over one aspect (previously defeating) of a person's life, generalizes remarkably to other aspects and sends the self-esteem in a spiral upwards. My own experiences in helping others change elements of their lives provide countless examples. The person who learns to stop biting her fingernails after 17 years of chewed cuticles alters her pride in how she dresses and who she talks to. Someone who takes control of a lifetime weight problem asks her boyfriend to marry her. The handicapped teenager who learns to file requests with his supervisor starts to ask shop assistants to help him find his way around the store. Social skills training programs can be planned to ensure the generalization of the clients' skills by examining the individual goals, and providing the resources for identifiable increments of success, no matter how small those increments may be.

CHAPTER 9

Children with Special Needs

In many respects, programs for handicapped children have much in common with the programs already described in this book. But there are also important differences; it is the purpose of this chapter to explore and clarify those differences. An interesting challenge arises with some populations: Their needs may give rise to special curricula (the skills of value are different) and at the same time they may require special approaches to teaching. Children who have special needs include, first, those with language disorders, and second, those deficient in basics, resulting from mental retardation, multiple (including physical) handicaps, or autism. Third, there are those who need extra skills because of visual or hearing impairment.

Public Law 94-142 (1975) has been in effect for a decade, bringing a far-reaching impact upon education for the handicapped. This law requires, essentially, that all children have access, through their school district, to the most effective and most suitable teaching programs available, thus maximizing the possibility of fulfilling their academic potential. In particular, mainstreaming has been implemented with considerable energy. Unfortunately, even where mainstreaming has enabled a handicapped child to catch up academically, there is evidence that the child seldom achieves social equivalence with nonhandicapped peers. Panzer, Wiesner, and Dickson (1978) claim that "children who are developmentally disabled are more often handicapped by lack of social skills than by intellectual limitations" (p. 406). There is also evidence

144

(Gresham, 1981) that handicapped children need to be *more* socially skilled to be rated as true peers with their nonhandicapped age-mates, and that mainstreaming has often exacerbated social adjustment problems for handicapped children. Despite the advances in educational opportunity, research and program development of social skills training for different types of handicap are very recent and sparse indeed.

LANGUAGE DISORDERS

Remarkably little consideration has been given to language disorders in social skills training. Perhaps because the field of speech and language therapy developed independently with its own specialized expertise, the two areas have been kept separate. Yet it is obvious that the social survival of children may frequently depend on the acquisition of basic language skills, and not just in cases of more severe problems such as mental retardation or autism. As a small beginning towards integrating these fields, the first section of this chapter will briefly review the treatment of stuttering. The development of functional language in autistic and severely retarded children is discussed later.

Stuttering

There is evidence to suggest that severe disorders of speech fluency have an organic origin. For example, stuttering runs in families, onset occurs 95% of the time by the age of 7 years, and 60% of the stutterers outgrow the disorder by adolescence. Although stuttering is demonstrably a problem of muscle tension, there exists an abundance of theories for what might cause the tension disorder. After many years of research and program development in this area, Ronald Webster (1980) has concluded that stuttering therapy requires an empirical, rather than a theoretically oriented, approach. The major elements of the treatment program, developed by Webster and others at Hollings College, Virginia, are described below.

Program for precision fluency shaping

This program consists of three 1-week phases, focusing on respiratory, phonatory, and articulatory responses, and their generalization to a wide variety of situations.

1a. Slow speech. Syllables are lengthened to match specific duration, under the control of diaphragmatic breathing. The control of respiration is taught using automated feedback of changes in the circumference of the rib cage.

1b. Gentle onset. Clients are taught to produce voicing with initially low-amplitude pulses, developing steadily to a normal volume, avoiding rapid changes in voice energy. Again technology assists, by providing immediate information descriptive of the acoustic speech signals. Gentle onset control can then be highly practiced for troublesome sounds.

2. Integration. The exaggerations above are moderated and integrated in articulation exercises. Functional speech, initially with short words only, becoming progressively more complex, provides the vehicle.

3. Generalization. Fluency skills are transferred to settings outside the clinic through a series of graduated exercises, beginning with short telephone calls.

Results of this program are impressive. It appears that 90% of their clientele (preschool children to mid-life adults) initially achieve fluency that puts them in the range of normal speakers. Studies providing 1-year follow-up data indicated only 10% regress to their pretreatment stuttering levels.

Webster emphasizes the empirical approach. That is, the sequence of functional changes is more important than the techniques used to achieve those changes. He also points to the importance of the intensity of therapy. If less than ten hours of training per week is provided, progress slows and dropping out increases. He concludes that therapy failures may be more often a product of inadequate application, rather than inappropriate methods – a conclusion similar to that reached in Chapter 2 with respect to the intensity of social skills training.

DEVELOPMENTAL DISABILITY

The popular adoption of the term *developmental disability* is a reflection of current thinking on the limitations of handicap. It implies, literally, that some forms of handicap are characterized by a limitation of development. In particular, mental retardation is viewed not so much as intellectual impairment but as a lowered capacity to mature. That is, the development of social, as well as intellectual, functioning can be expected to be "normal," *except that it takes longer to occur.* Under circumstances of nonintervention, therefore, many living skills are never learned. However, it is now widely agreed that for most people classified as "mentally retarded," skills for normal functioning can be acquired, if sufficient opportunities to learn are provided.

Autism and some forms of physical handicap may also be usefully construed as developmental disabilities. It is valuable in the present context, however, to consider sensory deficits separately. Children with visual or hearing impairments require help with special, compensatory skills, rather than basic skills. Thus, we are concerned in this section with children for whom there are delays or limitations in the acquisition of normal, adaptive social functioning.

Special programs are necessary for the developmentally disabled. Physical handicaps narrow the repertoire of activity, and intellectual handicaps prevent progress in natural situations in which social learning may take place. Once social delay has occurred, the condition perpetuates itself. That is, the chronological age of an 8-year-old mentally retarded boy advances him out of the milieu in which learning to function socially as a 4-year-old (the boy's mental age), normally occurs. The adaptation that the environment is programmed to teach becomes increasingly out of reach, and he is able to participate less and less. Inevitably, the physically handicapped person is also less able to participate; even given wheelchair access, the girl with spina bifida still cannot dance. People react differently to handicapped children, but the result is usually either to pamper or to neglect. In either case, the development of independent functioning is lost; to pamper is to remove the immediate need for independence, and to neglect is to provide too big a hurdle for the development of autonomy.

Considerations for Training

Specific considerations emerge from descriptions of successful programs for training mentally retarded people in communication skills. These differences do not suggest major changes to the basic format, style, or content of social survival training as described elsewhere in this book. But they do imply important minor modifications.

Most obviously, it must be expected that training take place more slowly. But it is important to recognize what takes the extra time. First, much more detail is required. Where the curriculum for two lessons expands into six, each component skill must be reanalyzed with *three times the detail.* It is not sufficient simply to spend three times as long training the more broadly defined skills identified in the curriculum for nonhandicapped children. For example, one strategy for making conversation with a stranger is to remark on some aspect of the present environment. This task can be further analyzed into observing major features of the environment (e.g., the room, the elevator), suggesting what can be said about it (e.g., the color, the delay), and practicing ways to phrase chosen comments.

Second, it is imperative that *learning takes place by doing.* It is, of course, generally true that skills are acquired more thoroughly and permanently when the training includes an experiential component. However, with high-functioning trainees a considerable amount will be acquired through explanation alone. But the lower the level of functioning, the less effective are the training components that do not involve the trainees in active participation. Therefore, the extra time spent on a more finely grained subdivision of tasks should be devoted primarily to activities such as imitation or rehearsal. For example, controlled studies of comparative procedures by Matson and others (Matson, 1982; Senatore, Matson, & Kazdin, 1982) show the addition of practice components to be most clinically significant. Although these results were obtained with mentally retarded adults, they are likely to apply even more definitely to children.

Third, there is some evidence for a preference of the visual medium, since it relies less on language. That is, it is better to provide a demonstrative role play than to try to describe a situation. There may be rewards from the greater initial effort to prepare pictures, slides, and videotapes for this population.

Finally, the curriculum chosen must be more basic. While this idea is obvious, many of the curriculum components may not be. Some of the fundamentals of communication are so basic that they are easily overlooked. For example, as adults we generally forget that we once *learned* to make what we say we did "correspond" to what we actually did. At an even more basic level, we learned to identify fundamental concepts and classifications, such as "motor vehicle" and "stranger." In extreme cases, these fundamentals need a training program of their own, as discussed in the subsequent sections of this chapter. In the immediately following section a program is described to address less basic, but nonetheless complex, handicaps.

Program Description: Multiply Handicapped Young Adults

The following program was developed by Marie Hood and me for the Auckland Crippled Children Society (CCS), and has been run by her and colleagues for several years. Our research studies have demonstrated the effectiveness of the program relative to a waiting list control condition, and the practical importance for the development of clients is perceived favorably by the staff of CCS.

The CCS facility includes sheltered workshops and vocational training for teenagers and young adults whose handicaps make it difficult for them to achieve social independence, and in particular, to compete in the open work force. The CCS staff found that even when trained with competitive vocational skills, their clients often lost or left jobs after very short periods of time. Independent on-site assessments usually cited the main reason as "social immaturity." The social skills program was developed, therefore, for clients in their mid-teens or a little older who had mild to severe developmental disabilities, but who were considered capable of eventually acquiring vocational skills acceptable to the marketplace. Some already had minimal exposure to trial work settings, and some had no current expectations for outside employment. All had basic oral language skills, although many had moderate speech difficulties.

The objectives of the program were to train basic conversational skills and assertiveness relevant to the handicapped population. The skills were applicable to friends of both sexes, workmates, and strangers. The situations included making friendships, using public services, applying for jobs, and dealing with criticism.

Program

Format. Clients were trained in groups with a maximum number of eight in each. Although people with disabilities require intensive training, the importance of peer modeling increases with severity of disability, so that individual training, perhaps surprisingly, is less efficient. The intensity of procedures and the frequent need to enact situations, however, requires two group leaders.

Each session was about 1 hour long; it was our experience that trying to work more than one and a quarter hours resulted in loss of concentration and energy. In most cases, the program consisted of six weekly sessions, plus before and after treatment meetings for assessment purposes. This time frame allowed the training of conversational skills and an introduction to assertiveness. In programs for more advanced clients, four additional sessions were provided to train job-related social skills (in particular, employment application interviews). A session-by-session outline follows (a manual with more detail is available on request).

Pre-assessment. Baseline levels of performance were assessed from three sources. General level of functioning was identified through questionnaires responded to by CCS staff and by the clients themselves. The group supervisor helped all clients to complete their self-assessments and to develop short- and long-term goals for treatment. Information from these questionnaires and goal statements was used to modify the curriculum of later sessions. The role-play exercises in session 1 were videotaped and also used for assessment purposes. The video recordings were scored on rating scales based on the specific components of social skills listed at the end of Chapter 1.

Session format. Each training session followed the format advocated in Chapter 2 for social skills training programs in general. That is, they involved discussion of "homework" assignments, role play, and other exercises to develop understanding and acquire skills, practice to criterion on prespecified items, use of modeling, rehearsal, feedback, positive reinforcement, video feedforward, and group discussion. Each session ended with homework assignments and announcements of the next session's topic.

Session 1: Introduction and overview. The concept of social skills is introduced as a way of getting along with people to gain self-confidence and independence. Common problems are identified (shyness, aggressiveness, difficulties in saying no or asking for help). These problems are seen as stemming from the trainees *giving up* too easily or *feeling inferior* to others around them. Therefore, it is explained that the program will teach participants how to be effective, and it will provide practice so that they will develop a sense of their own effectiveness (cf. self-efficacy, Bandura, 1977a). Clients first experience seeing themselves on video by being recorded while they introduce themselves (to people they already know). Tapes are replayed immediately with positive comments only. Each trainee then pulls a topic from a hat and attempts a 2-minute impromptu talk (e.g., the local Special Olympics). Even when the youths have poor speech abilities, drawing items out of a hat generates a lottery atmosphere, which engenders a general sense of fun. These talks are recorded (but not replayed) to complete the pre-assessment data collection. The session ends with a brief introduction to non-verbal messages, with an assignment to watch television at home with the sound off "to see if you can understand it."

Session 2: Nonverbal communication. Videotapes from the previous week (self-introductions) can be edited between sessions to show 1 minute of good communication for each client. This serves as a reminder of previous work and tends to boost energy and morale for the current session. An imaginary box with imaginary objects is "handed around" to promote discussion of nonverbal communication. The function of eye contact is identified, and the trainers role-play good and bad examples for group discussion. These discussions lead into exercises of nonverbal expression of emotion. Individuals explore, in pairs, facial expression, hand gestures, body posture, and voice tone, volume, and inflexion, with emphasis on the expressive aspect of communication (perception and reception easily follow). These exchanges are videotaped. If time allows, the best examples are replayed, emphasizing the successful aspects (e.g., "You see how she smiled when you looked at her, right in the eye") for immediate feedforward. At the end of the session individual assignments are made for the practice of nonverbal expression. The topic of the next session is anticipated by a brief reference to nonverbal signs that indicate one person's interest in hearing the other person speak.

Session 3: Interpreting conversational cues. The session begins with one-minute, edited versions of the best performances of each participant from the week before. The group is immediately divided into pairs, and all individuals are given a picture of a piece of furniture. One individual in each pair describes his or her picture without naming it. The other asks questions and tries to guess what it is; then roles are reversed. The best examples of video recordings of these exchanges are replayed to illustrate showing interest and handing over conversation. Specific features are identified (e.g., posture, smiles, mutual gaze, changes in voice inflexion). Specific role plays are set up (again in pairs) for social situations based on individual goals for treatment previously identified. Clients are encouraged to display (deliberately) both positive and negative examples of showing interest and handing over. Video recordings are immediately replayed only for the successful, positive examples. The week's assignment is to start a conversation with someone not known very well. Each group member is helped to identify the specific circumstances in which this assignment might take place, and is asked to make a record of how long the conversation is sustained. The next week's topic is identified.

Session 4: Starting conversations. Feedforward vignettes from the previous session are reviewed and the homework assignment discussed. Three skills are addressed: open-ended questions, attention to free information, and answering questions. The first two are demonstrated by the group leaders and then practiced by the group in pairs in the format of guessing games. The third skill, answering questions, is first demonstrated in terms of using and giving free information, and then practiced by the group. Exchanges of all three skills are videotaped and the best examples replayed immediately: essentially the ability to pick up on topics of mutual interest and to avoid either inviting or giving yes/no answers. The homework assignment is to start conversations with open-ended questions.

Session 5: Maintaining conversations. Video recordings edited from the last week's exercises are reviewed along with the homework assignments. A further three skills are introduced, built on the skills previously learned. These are: breaking into a conversation, changing the topic, and terminating conversation. In all cases role plays are constructed around situations recalled from recent events in the lives of the participants. The circumstances are reconstructed and the exchanges are improved. For example, in front of "I have to go, I'll miss my bus," add "It's been great talking to you," and disengage with nonverbal cues. Role plays are acted out, rotating the active group membership, with others looking on. Again, video can be used for feedforward. The week's assignment is to join a conversation and report on how it was achieved.

Session 6: Special situations–assertiveness. Video feedforward and the assignments are reviewed. This meeting is the last training session in the introductory series. It is common for clients to need a consolidation period or even to recycle through the introductory sessions before proceeding to the advanced training series.

The primary purpose of this session is to distinguish between passive, assertive, and aggressive responses (see Chapter 1; also Alberti & Emmons, 1974; Lange & Jakubowski, 1976). Assertiveness is defined not as a means to get one's own way, but as a means to express positive or negative feelings without guilt and embarrassment. The group leaders role-play illustrations of passive, aggressive, and assertive behavior, pointing out the nonverbal and verbal elements practiced in previous sessions. Three rules for assertive behavior are identified: be direct; be spontaneous; be honest.

Two assertive skills are practiced by all group members. The first is the distinction between "I messages" and "you messages." The second is the principle of escalation. That is, even when annoyed it is better to start by being minimally assertive. However, one should also have the skill to escalate the demand quality of assertive expression when it is needed. Assertiveness is rehearsed in the group to four levels of escalation. Again video is used to provide examples of the best role plays. The homework assignment for all participants is to find situations in which "I statements" can effectively replace accusatory remarks. For some participants, situations for escalating assertion can be identified.

Post-assessment. The group meets again for half an hour to repeat the exercises of session 1 (introductions and 2-minute impromptus), which are videotaped for subsequent analysis. The other half of the hour is used for completion of self-report questionnaires and supervisor report data, including a re-examination of treatment goals. Sometimes a group outing to a restaurant, requiring generalization of many of the skills learned in the program, is appropriate.

Sessions 7 through 10: Advanced skills. Reviews of edited video recordings and homework assignments are conducted at the beginning of each session. The overall objective of this series is to develop self-presentation skills for the preparation of job applications and taking an interview. Skills covered include:

- preparation of resumé, completion of Labor Department forms
- self-description of disability in positive terms (what trainee *can* do, not what he or she cannot do)
- identify available job openings, rewrite resumé
- role-play telephone enquiry, meeting the secretary
- planning appearance, punctuality, initial impression (trainees come to this session as if it were their actual job interview)

Role-play interview opening, responding to challenge, being positive about disability, enthusiasm, closing, and calling back.

These sessions are useful only to those old enough and able enough to contemplate unsheltered employment. Further details can be found in the training manual available from the authors, or in books focusing on adult issues.

Correspondence Training

A procedure of particular value to training social skills with a developmentally disabled population has been dubbed *correspondence training*. The term refers to the correspondence between words and action. The procedure was developed originally with young, normally functioning children (Risley & Hart, 1968). But its particular value in the present context is as an example of teaching a *communication response class* that is usually acquired during normal development, but may need to be specifically taught to low functioning children.

The response class in question, more exactly, is the correspondence between what a child *does* and what the child later *reports having done*. In very young children (preschool), a large discrepancy between these two events is normal. This discrepancy is not to be seen as dishonesty or memory failure. Simply understood, the verbal response is under the control of the immediate context (predominantly the child's perception of what was right to do), rather than under the control of his or her memory. In early stages of development, what children say they did corresponds more closely to what they say they *will* do than to their actual behavior.

Classic studies in this training procedure addressed community consequence issues, such as littering (Chapman & Risley, 1974). In these studies it was found that before going into the playground children, when asked, would state their belief that the appropriate place for food wrappings and such was the litter basket, and that is where they would put them. In the playground, however, the children dropped litter mostly on the ground. When asked afterwards what they did with their wrappings, they would report putting them in the litter baskets. The discrepancy was quite easily eliminated by providing corrective feedback from observed information ("You did put one wrapper in the trash, but you dropped three pieces on the ground"). These studies produced the interesting finding that it was the playground behavior that changed to match the verbal responses, rather than the reverse. Studies of different kinds of self-care and recreational activities using correspondence training have confirmed that this type of correspondence is a response class. That is, the child learns to use verbal report to reflect more accurately the memory of what she or he did; the correspondence then readily generalizes to verbal report in other contexts, beyond the situation trained.

In general, learning to make more accurate correspondences between saying and doing is no doubt useful to social functioning. It avoids imputations of lying, for instance. But where the social survival of the child, rather than the ecology of the playground, is of primary concern, there are training targets more suitable than littering. Few such targets have so far been explored. One good example is learning to share and praise through correspondence training (Rogers-Warren & Baer, 1976). Self-control (Karoly & Dirks, 1977) is relevant. In fact, Risley (1977) considers the most important contribution of correspondence research to be its implications for the concept of self-control. He suggests an equivalence between self-control and word-deed correspondence: "When a person exhibits a problem relating to lack of self-control, this problem can be interpreted as resulting from the absence of predictable informed audiences in his normal life with whom to discuss his affairs and ambitions, and/or to a weak general relationship between his words and his deeds" (p. 80).

Some of the earliest (Risley & Hart, 1968) and some of the latest studies (Baer, Williams, Osnes, & Stokes, 1984) have targeted toy play. However, these have focused on toy selection and generalization, most frequently (by happenstance) resulting in solitary play (e.g., beads, books). The latter studies were not designed out of concern for social functioning, so these remarks suggest no criticism. Rather the excellence of these studies in demonstrating the versatility and effectiveness of correspondence training reminds us that this intervention procedure is, at present, considerably underused. The broader application to social concerns of children is promisingly wide open for exploration.

It is also clear that the application of correspondence training to other populations is also underexplored. In particular, children with developmental disability can benefit from this technique. Most applications thus far have been with preschool children (see Karlan & Rusch, 1982). The choice of preschoolers has presumably rested on their readiness to learn this response class. Clearly, children chronologically older but of equivalent mental age because of developmental delays would be as appropriate. Again, this wider application simply awaits practitioners with the priorities to pursue it.

Autism and Severe Mental Retardation

When disabilities become more extreme, qualitative differences emerge in the considerations for communication training. Some of these differences concern processes that occur spontaneously and at a reasonably adaptive rate in other children, but that must be programmatically taught to very low functioning children (e.g., generalization). Beyond these considerations are processes that seem to operate quite differently in profoundly handicapped children, such as a preference for sign language. The most important of these special considerations and the appropriate training procedures are discussed in the sections following.

First, a word of clarification on the populations to be addressed. Autism is very distinct from mental retardation. Some autistic children appear highly intelligent with respect to certain functions; generally, IQ's, as measurable, are in the retarded range, but appear in the normal range subsequent to treatment. Characteristics that distinguish autism include a high rate of ritualistic behavior (e.g., hand flapping), destructive, and self-injurious behavior. Whereas these activities are antisocial, autism is mostly distinctly set apart by its *asocial* nature: very little attachment to people, and absent or abnormal speech (see Lovaas, 1977 for a thorough description; see Krug, Arick, & Almond, 1980 for a behavior checklist distinguishing autism from other disorders). Much of the treatment for autistic children depends first on overcoming or avoiding the problems raised by their lack of interest in or response to social interaction. In other aspects, successful interventions for autism have much in common with those for severely retarded children. Both populations pose enormous challenges to social skills trainers.

Generalization. Two distinct abilities may be seen to constitute generalization: Generalization across situations refers to having the same response to *different contexts* and generalization of behavior refers to the making of *different* but functionally similar *responses* in a given context. *Discrimination* is the process that keeps generalization in check, on the basis of critical features held in common by the various situations or responses. For example, a child may learn to hug his mother. The situation that prompts a hug may generalize to other family members, to strangers, to the dog, and to creatures that move. The behavior may generalize to smiles, kisses, "hello, I love you" and other forms of greeting and affection. Discrimination allows the child to avoid 12-year-olds who do not like to be kissed or crocodiles with a taste for young children.

Adaptive generalization as a response class cannot be taken for granted, as cogently pointed out by Stokes and Baer (1977), and is of special concern for autistic and severely mentally retarded children (see Baer, 1981; Carr, 1980). Successful training techniques involve first ensuring that one response in one situation is thoroughly learned, and then gradually introducing more and more variation into all aspects of the training. The context can and should be varied by altering the physical setting (different rooms, outside vs. inside, home vs. school), the other people or objects present (sometimes a specific object, such as a teddy bear, can be taken from one setting to another to begin generalization training and then faded out), the time of day, and sensory conditions, such as lighting, smells, and background noise. Different trainers can be used, verbal components worded differently, and a variety of models employed. Different consequences and variable delay intervals can be used and reinforcements given less frequently and for a greater variety of responses. The greater the number of variations during training, the greater the probability of further generalization occurring.

Concept acquisition offers an important example of generalization. One cannot teach social interaction appropriate to strangers, for example, unless the child has a concept of "stranger." As Carr (1985) has pointed out, concepts are not readily formed by autistic children. He cites evidence (e.g., Hupp & Mervis, 1982) that certain exemplars ("prototypes") are better than others in the training of concept formation. Unfortunately, there is no "ready reckoner" of ideal exemplars for all possible concepts. But I would venture to guess that an *appreciation of stereotypes* will provide a useful beginning. For example, a stereotypical stranger may be a man in his 20s, wearing coat and hat, walking, looking at signposts. Another may be a graying woman in a tour bus. Training with carefully selected exemplars will speed up the process of concept acquisition.

Expression versus reception. For most children in the early stages of language acquisition, the ability to understand precedes the ability to express. That is, a 2-year-old child who expresses herself in two word sentences may perfectly well comprehend an adult who speaks to her in complex grammatical form and with a vocabulary beyond that ever heard from the child herself. This priority seems logical and fortunate for language to be learned in a natural environment. Therefore, we might logically expect to teach language-retarded individuals according to the same priority.

However, it seems that for individuals who have severe language retardation, expression precedes reception (Cuvo & Riva, 1980). These children learn faster if they are first taught to express new words or grammatical forms. Their comprehension readily follows. Part of the reason for the switch in sequence is probably a function of motor development. The expressiveness of a 2-year-old with normal language development is impeded by the slow development of articulation. An older child with language difficulties will be comparably superior in the development of the motor coordination required for speech.

This finding underscores the importance of involving the clients in action for optimal learning. Highly intelligent children sometimes learn quite well while passive and uninvolved (e.g., reading, listening). However, active engagement makes for better learning, a fact that becomes more imperative the lower the mental functioning of the child. The principle of active engagement should not be confined to formal teaching sessions, but can be used to design a productive learning environment.

One simple and effective way to achieve this effect is to make language *functional* by presenting linguistic barriers between the child and what she or he wants (see Carr, 1985; Risley & Twardosz, 1976). Toys, food, and other desired items can be visible but inaccessible without asking for permission or assistance. In most homes and institutions these items are provided with maximum access or even given to children who are reluctant to take them. This environment is appropriate to enable children to sample and to acquire an interest, but once a reasonable engagement level has been achieved, this system works against the development of communication.

Sign language. All language is symbolic, and it is a mistake to assume that the commonly spoken words are necessarily the best symbols for all people. Admittedly, the natural evolution of spoken language ensures that the spoken word of a given culture is efficient and most easily mastered by the majority of individuals in that culture. But for a minority of handicapped individuals, a completely different set of symbols may be far more accessible. It seems that many children who are severely mentally retarded or autistic grasp sign language (devised for the deaf) more readily than oral language (Poultin & Algozzine, 1980). In certain cases, some other symbolic system may prove easier to learn (such as pointing at pictures; see Fristoe & Lloyd, 1978).

Sign or picture language, and other more universal non-verbal communications, can then be used to extend conventional oral skills. If oral speech routinely accompanies signing, the latter may be gradually faded out. The acquisition of oral language in this way seems particularly promising with echolalic children. When a child who wants help to go to the bathroom tugs an adult's hand, this can be seen as an appropriate non-verbal communication of the child's need. This type of situation provides optimal circumstances for the teaching of conventional language, as described in the following section.

Incidental teaching. The principle of maximizing learning, by adding it to a situation in which the child is already voluntarily engaged, is called *incidental teaching*. It seems ideally suited to conditions of extreme language retardation, although most of the research so far has been with culturally disadvantaged preschoolers (Hart & Risley, 1975, 1982).

For example, a child may want to play with a spinning top. Whether the child just points and says "uh!" or asks politely and articulately, there is an opportunity to elaborate on the associated language. The supervising adult can model the word "top" or ask which color, large or small. Actually handing over the top or helping to make it spin then acts as very meaningful reinforcement for the child's attempts at using language. Not only do children learn more, it has been found that children prefer supervisors who use incidental teaching over those who do not. A compelling case, with empirical backing, has recently been proposed by McGee, Krantz, and McClannahan (1985) for the use of incidental teaching with autistic and other children with severe language impairment.

Following is a synopsis of procedures, adapted from Hart and Risley (1978). They emphasize first, making the child's language functional (i.e., it helps him to get what he wants) and second, working only in response to the child's initiation (initiations can generally be construed as requests of some type).

Engagement.
1) Focus all attention on the child.
2) Clarify the child's initiation if too ambiguous (e.g., "Do you want a toy?") to enable elaboration, as indicated below.
   Elaboration. The strategies for elaborating on the child's initiating interaction depend on the type of request.
3) Requests for materials or permission. This initiation lends itself to more demanding tasks, such as the development of grammar (because the child's interest in satisfying the request is naturally high). For example, McGee and colleagues, cited above, taught prepositions, mostly in this context ("You want the box *where?*" requiring "in front of," "next to," etc., and quietly insisting on a verbal response).
4) Seeking approval or attention. Respond with "tell me what else you can do," or "so tell me, what is that you're playing with?" Do not correct the approval-seeking child in this context, even if she is wrong, but continue the elaboration.
5) Requests for assistance. When the child seems to be seeking a procedure, a task analysis is required. Break down the procedure into very small steps. Tell the child the first one, and say, "Now you tell me what you can do next." If the task analysis is fine enough, the next step will be obvious.

6) Enquiries for information. Make an indirect response so that the child collaborates on finding the answer (e.g., "Where would we find out about that?").
Help. The elaboration should be brief and lead the child promptly to satisfying the request. Quite likely he will need assistance.
7) Prompt or hint at the answer. "The horse is pulling the c_ _ _."
8) Model the response if it is not forthcoming after a prompt. "This color is green; what color is this?"
Closure.
9) If all else fails, instruct the child directly with the functional response: "Can you say 'green'?" This instruction ensures that the interaction ends on a positive note.
10) Finally, confirm for the child, with enthusiasm, that she was right, and some aspect of what she said was right. "That's great, you are right; the doll is *inside* the box!"

Overall, the interactions work best when kept brief and varied. Given the manner in which incidental teaching develops language as functional to the trainee's own purposes, and it takes place in context and with brevity, its usefulness with a severely disabled population is self-evidently promising.

Curriculum. In his excellent chapter on behavioral approaches to language training with autistic children, Edward Carr (1985) points to the importance of curriculum development – the content of communication training. Whereas the methodology of how to do the training with these populations has made considerable progress over the last one or two decades, the question of what to train has not received the same attention. He suggests that the contributions of psycholinguists to information on language acquisition provide a potential basis for curriculum development. This possibility, however, remains very much to be explored by those who devise communication training programs for children with severe handicaps.

As a brief illustration of the importance of curriculum, consider teaching an initial functional vocabulary to a child. Reichle and Keogh (1985) have lucidly pointed out the complications in a seemingly simple vocabulary of "drink," "orange juice," and "milk" (advocated by others). The child faces the conceptual hurdle that both juice and milk are subclasses of drink. What is worse, drink is both a noun and a verb.

Carr has made the interesting suggestion that it is sometimes useful to view behavior problems as forms, albeit socially unacceptable, of communication (a view similar to that held by some family systems theorists; see Gurman and Kniskern, 1981). Thus, he suggests that problems, such as tantrums or aggression, and even self-injury, may be expressions of frustration or other emotions for which the child has a very limited expressive repertoire (Carr & Durand, 1985). The most positive approach, then, is to use these events as opportunities to teach appropriate social skills. However, the biggest challenge of autism remains: Children with this affliction use minimal communication to meet their physiological personal needs, and appear to find no intrinsic value in social exchange.

SENSORY AND PHYSICAL IMPAIRMENT

Children who have impaired sight or hearing, or who suffer focused neurological or physical disabilities without loss of overall intellectual functioning, differ from those children already discussed. Those with sensory or physical impairment generally need not basic skills but extra skills to compensate for the disability. Children with handicaps experience two disadvantages. First, there are some unique forms of social exchange necessitated by the handicap (e.g., a request for help where there is no wheelchair access), which they will not observe among their ablebodied peers. Second, any handicapped person needs to be slightly *more* socially skilled to be rated on a par with a nonhandicapped person. These considerations will slightly alter the curriculum and the frequency of social skills training endeavors with this population.

Notwithstanding the attention to social needs provided by those working in settings with children with sensory impairments, very few reports have been published, and those only in the last few years. Generally, the reported findings are from applications of established training techniques to this population, or they are investigative studies. For example, Farkas, Sherick, Matson, and Loebig (1981) used role play and differential reinforcement of appropriate behavior to eliminate what appeared to be schizophrenic manifestations in a 12-year-old blind girl.

Two other studies reporting intervention with *visually impaired* children bear describing. Van Hasselt, Hersen, Kazdin, Simon, and Mastantuono (1983) worked with four totally blind adolescent girls. They provided the components of training as generally advocated — information, modeling, role play, feedback — over 3 or 4 weeks, five sessions a week, 15 to 30 minutes per session, with a curriculum of posture, gaze, voice tone, and making requests. In contrast to programs for other children, this one emphasized verbal prompts and manual guidance. The

multiple baseline analysis (across behaviors) provided good support for
the efficacy of the program. Ruben (1983) adapted assertiveness training paradigms for the blind and partially sighted. He had 13 slightly
older clients (15 to 40 years) and the curriculum included issues concerning discrimination against blind people. Adaptations to the procedure
for the clientele included more attention to description, emphasis on the
meaning of vocal tone, and "gestural prompting" (although it is not clear
what was meant by this term). Generalization was achieved by training in settings providing different (nonvisual) sensory cues (e.g., the
cafeteria vs. dormitories).

Recently, Matson and colleagues (1986) investigated assessment instruments and basic social functioning with a sample of visually impaired people (75 subjects, ages 9 to 22 years). They found a high similarity between adolescent self-report and rating by their teachers,
suggesting an ability of this group to perceive themselves as others see
them. Very curiously, in a comparison between 45 visually handicapped
children and a nonhandicapped group, they found more inappropriate
social skills (of the impulsive type) with the nonhandicapped.

I have found a very few reports directly addressing the social skills
of *hearing impaired* young people. Kusche, Garfield, and Greenberg
(1983) investigated the emotional and social attributions of deaf teenagers. They found that the level of language development was the most
highly significant contributor to the accurate perception of social situations and the emotional components. Overall, they found that deaf
17-year-olds had an equivalent perception to hearing children of only
6 years. The area clearly invites intervention and further research.

A social skills training program for teenagers with severe hearing impairments has been developed by Smith, Schloss, and Schloss (1984).
They reported working with five 17 to 18-year-olds, described as having social or emotional disorders. They were all fluent in Signed English,
but variable in other language capacities. In many respects the social
skills training program had objectives and a format similar to other programs (conversation, questions, criticisms, and compliments; 30 minute
sessions, three times a week). However, a major point of difference for
this program was the use of a table game, in place of the scene-setting
element, to raise the social interaction issues. The game used playing
cards, on which the interaction issue and a prompt were written; for example, "You just spilled your soda in the lunchroom and need a mop.
You say . . . . " (p. 9). Although the game is competitive (it has a "win-
ner"), it is divided into sections that require all players to finish, thus
also encouraging cooperation. It seems likely, therefore, that some

brainstorming and peer modeling would take place. Other elements typical of social skills training – trainer modeling, rehearsal, corrective feedback, positive reinforcement, and assignments – were incorporated into each session.

In a total of 38 sessions, all trainees reached criteria built into the card game (a valuable asset of this approach, it seems). Smith and colleagues then found clear evidence of the benefits of training, as measured in structured role plays and assessments in the natural environment. General comments offered by other staff associated with the program, and the enthusiasm expressed by the participating teenagers confirm the promise of this program.

A few programs for *physically disabled* people have been reported in the literature. In 1984 Starke could find only four studies "which have evaluated the effectiveness of assertiveness of social skills training with physically disabled subjects" (p. 3), and added two of her own, in which trainees improved their assertiveness and also their self-perceptions. None of these reported programs was for children, however. Most served young university students; one was for disabled war veterans.

A review chapter entitled "Social Skills and Physical Disability" (Dunn & Herman, 1982) is also totally oriented to adults. It identifies two major areas of special concern to this population: employment issues and status relationships. The first of these is relevant to older teenagers (see program for multiply handicapped earlier in this chapter). The second area, that of status relationships, is relevant to young children of all ages. In this area, the population-specific issues are most frequently those of asking for help when it is needed and turning help down when it is not needed. The authors have developed a "Spinal Cord Injury Assertion Questionnaire" (p. 124) to measure subjective discomfort in situations such as: "Ask somebody to help you empty your leg bag," and, "Tell a friend that it is difficult for you to accept the amount of help that he gives you." To devise a program for physically disabled children, a relevant curriculum would seem to be the most important innovation. The issues raised by Dunn and Herman provide a useful place to begin.

Overall it appears that the children with sensory and physical handicaps are underresearched and less than understood. In particular, they would seem to be able to benefit crucially from social skills training, and very few people have tried, or at least, reported their attempts.

CHAPTER 10

Teenagers

As children get older they change, and so does their environment. The teen years bring the most interesting and dramatic changes. For the first time since starting school, the adolescent experiences growth that is qualitatively different, not just a bigger and better version of what was before. New quantities of hormones affect the personality as well as the body, and not too subtle differences occur in the values given to aspects of the environment (hence, the iniquitus "peer pressure"). In this chapter, the important developmental differences that contribute to social skills (and their deficits) will be reviewed. The arising problems and their management will be discussed with particular attention to juvenile delinquency.

DEVELOPMENT

Adolescence is a period of life frequently bestowed with romantic description—but never by those who are themselves adolescents, or are currently attempting to live with any. In his engaging synopsis of *Adolescence*, J. C. Conger (1979) quotes Samuel Butler: "Like spring an overpraised season—delightful if it happens to be favoured, . . . but . . . more remarkable, as a general rule, for biting east winds than genial breezes." It is a time of most rapid changes in *physique, intellect*, and *sexuality*. These changes are matched by radically emerging *social prior-*

ities, through which the young person struggles towards an *adult identity*. Some discussion of these issues is provided in this section.

The *organismic* changes that take place are scarcely short of a biological revolution. The growth spurt will result in five or even ten inches of added height, and most of it will probably occur in a single year. But that could be any year of age between 10 and 17. Other physical changes (e.g., the deepening of a boy's voice, the girl's emerging figure of womanhood) remain unpredictable throughout adolescence, providing the youth with years of uncertainty. No little flag pops out, as with a roast turkey, to say, "I am done now." But the resulting adult body image sets the limits to be lived with for decades to come. Therefore, the nature and timing of these developments affect the social being. Will I ever stop growing? Will I always have pimples? Am I simply abnormal? To be reassured of normalcy, it is necessary to conform; but the greatest need for conformity comes when it is least possible. Either early or late maturation presents problems for adolescents, but the disorders of late maturation are most likely to persist in adulthood (Rogers, 1985) — perhaps because of failures in sports and dating activities.

Intellectual growth is almost as rapid (see Keating, 1980 for a review). In our teenage years our perceptual and analytical capabilities reach their peak of capacity and flexibility. The major qualitative shift in thinking style pointed out by Piaget is the sudden development of ability to comprehend the abstract, in particular the future — a shift of concern from the real to the possible. Whereas the younger child may use an imaginary world to embellish the present reality, a teenager can see the present as serving the future or in comparison with current alternatives. Thus, an adolescent's own family start to come under criticism, as do other systems of which the young person is a part. In 99% of cases these criticisms are theoretical exercises, explorations of newly discovered mental powers, rather than a physical threat to family or country (Conger, 1979). Adults and adolescents who recognize this activity for what it is can respond positively to the new form of social exchange.

The teenage ability to wrestle with the future and other abstractions combines with the insecure body image, adding to a preoccupation with the search for a sense of identity: Who am I? What will I be? The questioning process may produce the exploration of many and varied goals. The resulting extremes, changeability, and downright contrariness can lead to family distress and sorely tested friendships. But again, if the behavior can be recognized as a necessary exploration of self-concept, it can be responded to productively. Communication is improved by accepting some bizarreness as a passing phase, and the readiness to explore alternative "selves" can be capitalized upon in social skills training.

With adolescent growth, the most obvious qualitative changes involve the increase in *sex differences*. Social interactions are made more complex by the teenager's search for identity, not just as an adult but as a man or as a woman. As testes and ovaries start to enlarge, boys and girls begin to take more notice of the opposite sex, experiencing both interest and apprehension. One of the linguistic developments at this time is the use of irony, in particular, *double entendre*. An apparent preoccupation with double meanings and sexual innuendo simply reflects the combination of a newfound analytic ability with an increase in hormones.

Prior to adolescence children will have had mostly same-sex friendships, often asserting some rivalry with the other sex. Adolescent boys' interest in girls, and vice versa, begins with a mixture of erotic undertones (or overtones). The transition into heterosexual society will be most smoothly achieved by adolescents in groups (dance halls, sports grounds). The numbers provide safety, exercising the lowest demand on interpersonal skills until familiarity with the opposite sex leads more naturally to closer social contact. There is evidence that girls, at least, who date too early, are disadvantaged in their social development as much as those who do not date at all (Conger, 1979). Problems of shyness of intimacy may persist for girls or boys who date very infrequently.

Boys experience more specific impulses than girls do with respect to their growing sexual feelings. However, this finding is a generalization, and there is currently evidence of a trend in girls towards more direct sexual expression or initiation (Stone & Church, 1984). The active pursuit of intimacy (with or without sexual activity) for any teenager may serve more than anything as reassurance of self and social worth, as the young person struggles to integrate his or her newfound sexuality with self-concept and personal values. The delicacy of these matters makes the ability to express one's thoughts openly and honestly of paramount importance—no matter how confused or controversial those thoughts may be. Seventy percent of parents do not discuss any major topics of sexuality with their teenage children, and it is this group of adolescents who register the highest rate of sexual experiences. This connection between parent-child communication and teenage sexual activity is purely correlational, but it is highly suggestive of the value of better ability to communicate. A willingness for dialogue could at least help to dispel the myths that are still rife amongst young people: for example, DeAmicis and colleagues (1981) found that 40% of a sample of teenage females who had had premarital sex without contraceptives did so because they believed that they could not get pregnant. Those who, nonetheless, do get pregnant, face high probabilities of divorce, social isolation, and economic and educational disadvantage (see review of this area by Schinke, 1984).

These new bonding patterns bring changes in *social priorities*. Closer individual friendships bring a deepening need for emotional support and a greater vulnerability to rejection. Peer pressure forces the adoption of at least the trappings of a subculture, reflected in language and social interaction. However, parents usually remain the greatest influence of basic values. This fact is very readily masked by the teenager's behavior, and parents can experience considerable, sometimes painful, estrangement. Adolescents in every age stubbornly struggle to develop their own views on major moral issues of God, love, war, and loyalty; and in today's society, conflicting pressures are more complex than ever before. In many cases the choices are largely abstract (teenagers are notoriously more exploratory in theory than in action). But attempts to improve moral values without explanatory communication will result in superficial and insecure responses to life's more complex challenges.

The use of drugs provides a good example of a situation in which adults play a much greater role than they realize (see review by Horan & Harrison, 1981). Over 10% of high-school seniors have tried codeine, morphine, or heroin without prescription. Fifty percent have experimented with marijuana, and as many admit to using alcohol every week. At the same time as this explosion in illicit drug use, there has been a boom of similar proportions in adult use of prescription drugs; for example, nearly twice as many major tranquilizers were prescribed in 1977 as in 1964. Horan and Harrison note "of all the psychosocial correlates of drug use, perhaps the most convincing are the relationships between the individual's use of drugs and the drug-taking behavior of peers, older siblings, and parents" (p. 293). They also report that unassertive college students are most likely to use drugs either habitually or never; the most assertive students are more likely to have experimented and left drugs alone.

Society's message, with advertising support, is loud and clear: if you don't feel right, put another chemical into your system. And teenagers, with their bodies, minds, and souls in transition, often do not feel right. There are important, occasionally life-preserving, contributions made by pharmaceuticals to certain medical conditions, and some understanding of their specific and limited role is necessary to avoid equating drugs with quality of life.

Neither the pressures to experiment, nor the fears and dangers of exposing the problem later can be avoided completely. But both can be greatly alleviated by keeping open all possible lines of communication. Adults need to be receptive, before or after the event, to talk about the precipitators – peer pressure, promises of mind expansion, escape from emotional distress – with concern for the individual.

As a consequence of the qualities of physical and mental growth, adolescence is primarily a period of transition. Most of the struggles are, in a sense, those between leaving childhood and *approaching adulthood*. Unfortunately, in Western society that transition is very unclear. There are no specific rites of passage through which we are suddenly labeled by ourselves and our social group as a "man" or a "woman." The characteristic unevenness of maturity in American youth is, essentially, encouraged. The growing teenager would be helped towards more consistent behavior if expectations were more consistently designated. If one day the 13-year-old is expected to take sole responsibility for the behavior and safety of 7-year-old twins, and the next day is countermanded on the length of her hair, the designations are very inconsistent. To allay this confusion, parents and other significant adults must provide more consistency, accompanied by reasonable explanations of personal limits, and the development of rights and responsibilities. Very often the only way for adults to sharpen their consistency and explanations is for the adolescent to seek that sharpening, and to do so with the best qualities of assertiveness that will gain a cooperative audience.

Too much about adulthood is a mystery. In the name of "respectibility" and "consideration" parents actively promote the deepest elements of that mystery. Sex, birth, and death are kept as private as possible; even work – certainly its most emotional moments – is usually kept hidden from view. When children become teenagers, parents may well be entering middle age with their own developmental crises, and are perhaps not the ideal models for children looking forward to their twenties. If what it is "really like" to be an adult cannot be observed, the only way it can be understood is by talking about it. There is and always has been a generation gap, but its divisiveness is greatly exaggerated; if surveys are to be believed, 90% of teenagers (boys and girls about equally) think highly of their parents. Correlational studies indicate that parents remain the single most important factor in the adjustment – successful or otherwise – of adolescents (Conger, 1979). Hostility, rejection, and neglect by parents are vastly represented in all types of adolescent problems, from dropping out of school, to prostitution, to violent robbery (Weisberg, 1985).

PREVENTING DELINQUENCY

In general, behavioral disorders of teenagers who come to the attention of clinics and, therefore, get classified, appear to belong under three broad classifications: withdrawal, aggression, and age-inappropriateness. All are contributed to by social skills deficits, but only the first two play a part in juvenile delinquency problems, which have not been addressed as such in earlier chapters of this book. (Juvenile delinquency is defined simply as the violation of criminal law by a minor.) Social withdrawal can be a factor in drug abuse, in prostitution, and in some deliberately antisocial acts such as arson and vandalism. Interpersonal aggression plays a more obvious role in violent crime.

Juvenile crime has been increasing at an alarming rate. In 1978 Uniform Crime Reports (1979) found that nearly half of all arrests for serious crimes in the United States were of people under the age of 18 years, and the rate continues to increase. Rehabilitation of convicted offenders is proving to be extremely difficult, as evidenced by the greater than 50% recidivism rate within the first year of release (Burchard & Lane, 1982). Clearly, prevention is better than cure.

Purpose of Delinquency

It is valuable to regard delinquency as serving a purpose for the teenager. The perspective here is that the offensive behavior provides a quality of life (described below), or else the teenager would not do it. Whereas the means of achieving the purpose are not legitimate, the purpose itself may be.

Delinquent acts may be seen as the resolution of fear, frustration, poverty, or boredom. The acts that lead to the alleviation of these unpleasant conditions are not approved by society. That is, preemptive aggression, vandalism, theft, and harassment produce unpleasantness for others who, naturally, object. The objection often leads to the formality of arrest. However, the antisocial acts achieve a desired purpose and, therefore, may be expected to recur.

One may compare this phenomenon with Patterson's (1982) description of the development of aggression. The conditions that an infant must resolve are the most basic versions of those listed above – hunger, thirst, fear, and curiosity. They are resolved in ways considered adaptive only at a very early stage of development. Hungry infants are encouraged to take whatever food they can get their hands on, with no expectations of a sense of property. Toddlers may smash constructions from building blocks or best pottery from grandmother to amuse themselves; adults generally organize their environments with these possibilities in mind. However, similar activities in an 18-year-old will be regarded as theft and vandalism.

It may be seen, therefore, that an antisocial adolescence will be the natural result of a failure to replace early adaptive behavior with socially appropriate alternatives. Or delinquency may have more recent roots, possibly beginning in teenage years, developing through similar principles. The teenager, partly through rapid and uneven development, discovers dissatisfactions and searches to resolve them. Solutions that work to satisfy a goal will be naturally and most powerfully reinforced. Success breeds repetition. Some of the solutions will infringe upon the rights of others in society and alternatives may fail to be learned.

Thus, in using a social skills training approach to delinquency, it is helpful to view the objectives of delinquent behavior as legitimate, but the means of achieving the objectives as not so. The approach is to identify the quality of life sought by the teenager and to train more acceptable ways of attaining it. These "more acceptable ways" are taught to the teenager as alternatives, in which he or she can operate by choice.

Skills Deficits

It is also valuable to anticipate the situations that are likely to present problems for teenagers. Any training program will necessarily be preceded by individual assessments to establish the specific target areas most pertinent to the participants. Such assessments are made more efficient by an understanding of common trouble spots.

One relevant source of information is the Adolescent Problems Inventory, derived from a careful study by Freedman, Rosenthal, Donahoe, Schlundt, and McFall (1978). First, they identified a large number of situations likely to precipitate problems, through a review of the literature on delinquency, examination of case files, and discussions with delinquent youth and the professionals who work with them. These youth and professionals ranked the suggested situations on the basis of both how common and how difficult they perceived them to be. The situations were then field-tested in the following manner. Ninety narratives were devised to present the situations to a mixture of subjects, including nondelinquents, delinquents, and a few adults who worked with them. The subjects then responded in role play. The role plays were evaluated by judges who rated the competency of each response. Forty-four items, along with multiple-choice responses for each situation, were retained for the inventory on the basis of these experiences. Freedman and her colleagues then established the inventory items' reliability and their value in discriminating between samples of delinquents and "good citizens." The delinquents were residents of a state correctional institution. Good citizens were selected from high schools by counselors as law-abiding, responsible, involved in activities beyond the school curriculum, and getting along well with others. All but two of the items were found to discriminate between the two groups. The original study was done with boys only, but has been replicated since with girls, producing similar results.

One situation is presented here to illustrate a narrative and its response choice (Freedman et al., 1978, p. 1452):

> It is 1:30 at night, and you're walking along a street near your home. You're on your way home from your friend's home, and you know it's after curfew in your town. You weren't doing anything wrong. You just lost track of time. You see a patrol car cruising along the street and you feel scared, because you know you can get into trouble for breaking curfew. Sure enough the car stops next to you, the policeman gets out, and he says, "You there, put your hands on the car. Stand with your feet apart." What do you say or do now?
> Score:
> 8 – Either the subject does it without saying anything or he asks a brief general question respectfully. Example: "What's wrong officer?" "Is something the matter?" *or* he explains honestly and convincingly where he was.
> 6 – The subject explains where he was, etc., but in a less assertive or less convincing manner. Example: "I just got out of Pete Jones's house. You can call him if you want to."
> 4 – No specific criteria – midway between responses 6 and 2.
> 2 – The subject is antagonistic or flippant or insolent.
> 0 – Either the subject hits the policeman *or* he runs away.

All narratives contain comparable detail. To indicate the essence of the 44 items on the inventory, the authors' summary descriptions are shown in Table 10.1. It is clear that almost all the situations identified are interpersonal (involving peer pressure, provocations, accusations,

TABLE 10.1
Summary of Situations in Adolescent Problems Inventory*

1. A male, peer, stranger deliberately bumps into you on the street.
2. Same as #1, plus he blames you.
3. A gym teacher picks on you, makes you do extra pushups.
4. A friend suggests buying booze illegally.
5. Your father tells you to stay home on Saturday night.
6. You want to break up with your girlfriend without hurting her.
7. The school principal threatens to suspend you for hassling a substitute teacher.
8. You come home late at night and your father is waiting up for you and is angry.
9. You are called names by some guy in the schoolyard.
10. Your mother tells you to put on decent clothes before leaving the house.
11. A friend wants you to deliver some drugs; he offers drugs and money in return.
12. You are stopped on the street by a policeman after curfew.
13. Your father wants you to stop seeing one of your male friends.
14. Another boy makes an insulting remark about your mother.
15. A friend suggests that you two steal a handgun from a discount store.
16. You back your car over the neighbor's trash can; he yells at you.
17. Your friend is upset because you dated a girl he likes.
18. You've been grounded. A friend urges you to sneak out of the house.
19. Your father gives you an ultimatum about getting your hair cut.
20. A policeman comes to your door and asks for you.
21. A teacher accuses you of writing obscene words on the walls in the men's room.
22. A friend suggests joy riding in a car with the keys left in it.
23. You run out of gas, get to work late, and get fired.
24. Your father gets upset when you ask to borrow the car.
25. A friend asks you to steal something for him from where you work.
26. While with a friend, your father angrily tells you to go clean up your room.
27. An older friend asks you to help hold up a gas station.
28. You want to ask the manager of a McDonald's for a job.
29. Your girlfriend offers you a joint at a party.
30. You ask a girl for a date and she says that her father won't let her go out with you.
31. A girl's father meets you at the door and says he won't let her go out with you.
32. Peers at school hassle you about your criminal record.
33. A job interviewer is biased by your criminal record.
34. A teacher hassles you about your criminal record.
35. You wake up in a bad mood.
36. You need more money, your parents can't give it to you, and you are too young for a regular part-time job.

(continued)

TABLE 10.1
(*Continued*)

37. You are bored and want some fun.
38. You are studying for a final exam. A friend wants you to go to a concert instead.
39. Your mother forbids you to see a friend again.
40. Your girl breaks up with you. You feel miserable.
41. You don't feel like delivering your paper route today.
42. You feel hopelessly lost in a geometry class.
43. You have a car and want something exciting to do.
44. Your mother hassles you about going to church.

*Reprinted from Freedman et al. (1978), with permission of the publisher, American Psychological Association.

dealing with authority, and personal frustrations). The complete inventory and instruction manual are available from Barbara J. Freedman, Wisconsin Division of Corrections.

Levels of Prevention

Training strategies and programs to be discussed in the balance of this chapter will be considered as essentially preventive. That is, even working with incarcerated juveniles, the future, not the past, must be changed; success will be measured by the rate of (or lack of) further offending. The levels of prevention will be described here in terms of four different target populations. This approach may be contrasted with Caplan's (1961) widely cited three-level concept of primary, secondary, and tertiary prevention. Caplan's concept of prevention at different levels within the development of a disorder (taken from the medical disease model) has theoretical and practical interest; the conceptual identification of different target populations as levels of prevention set out below appears to have additional pragmatic advantages.

The levels are identified as follows; ironically, each lends itself to clear medical analogies:

1) In treatment. The prevention of recidivism may be compared with typical medication, or lifestyling prescriptions for heart attack patients. Pills do not cure the heart attack, which is now past, but they can prevent another. Psychological programs at this level are called rehabilitation.

2) At risk. A subpopulation may be identified as having a high likelihood of susceptibility in one of two ways: Risk may be induced by *location*. For many decades, smallpox was inoculated against, but, only for those entering an infected area; living in the inner city adds statistically to a child's risk of delinquency. Risk may also be recognized by *behavioral precursors*. Tetanus shots are typically given to people who have cut themselves; dropping out of classes is correlated with greater likelihood of delinquent arrest.

3) Whole population. In societies with high standards of medical care, all babies are given diphtheria inoculations. A society with high standards of preventive psychology would have social skills training as part of the elementary school standard curriculum.

4) Next generation. Even given the extent to which weight disorders may be genetically influenced, there is much that can be done by overweight parents to provide and encourage a healthier lifestyle for their children. The provision of parenting training for all the above levels of target population could provide the greatest long-term measure of prevention.

GROUP PROGRAMS AND STRATEGIES

Reviewers paint a gloomy picture of the effects of detention centers on juveniles. The search for optimism seems increasingly headed towards prevention in general (Graziano & Mooney, 1984, pp. 144–186), and social skills training in particular (Burchard & Lane, 1982; Spence, 1983).

Institutions

Overall, penal institutions have failed to dent the recidivism rate or to serve as a deterrent to the increasing number of new offenders. Burchard and Lane (1982) understate their view of long-term effects as "discouraging," pointing to a decade of rehabilitation programs that have either been abandoned or report 60% recidivism. Stumphauzer (1981) concluded "the situation is not going to get better; it is going to get worse." However, these reviewers were not without optimism for change. Much has been learned about the more productive attitudes with which to treat delinquent youth, and the short-term effects of intervention are highly positive. These findings suggest that the training methods are suitable, but we have yet to identify adequate targets for intervention or effective methods for maintenance of change.

Two general strategies seem to emerge from the suggestions of these reviewers. One is the concept of task-sentencing in the place of time-sentencing. This concept is not confined to restitution ("you will be discharged when you've finished repairing the vandalism you created"), but characterizes performance generally as the key exit criterion to sentencing. Criterion performance could include demonstration of skills proven to be correlated with low recidivism. The other strategy suggested is, indeed, a concentration on the training of more specific skills. The skills cited most frequently are academic, vocational, and interpersonal.

The particular interpersonal skills warrant close attention. Assertiveness training has been advocated, but the recommendation is not simple. Hull and Hull (1983) studied small but carefully balanced samples of offenders and nonoffenders (16 years of age, nine males and nine females in each group). They found differences in aggressiveness, but not in assertiveness. On the basis of their findings they recommended a focus on specific situations, not general assertiveness, especially in dealing with authority. Particularly for male offenders, they pointed to an excess of aggression, not a deficit of assertion.

Assessment

As described in Chapter 2 and elsewhere in this book, assessment is necessary both to evaluate the impact of the program (how many children improved, how much did they improve by, how cost-beneficial is the program) and to elucidate the specific skills deficits to be incorporated into the curriculum.

The first objective can be addressed by standardized questionnaires, role plays, and behavioral observations. Questionnaires to be recommended include the Adolescent Problems Inventory (API) already described, and the Children's Assertiveness Behavior Scale (CABS; see Michelson et al., 1983). The CABS is not designed specifically for the delinquent population, but has the advantage that a parallel form can be used by a supervisor to identify discrepancies between self-report and an observer's point of view (see Chapter 5). The API could easily be adapted for this purpose also. (Discrepancies occur at a low frequency, but when they do occur, they are usually important.) Another assessment instrument for adolescents is provided by Goldstein et al. (1980). However, this is designed solely for use by an informant and contains

50 items, which makes it likely to be unpopular when one supervisor has to respond for 10 or 20 youths. A sample item is as follows:

Apologizing: Does the youngster tell others that he/she is sorry after doing something wrong?   1   2   3   4   5
Problem situation: _____

The numbers 1 through 5 represent *never, seldom, sometimes, often, always*. The "problem situation" refers to any situation that is seen to present particular difficulty to the teenager.

A case can be made for developing one's own assessment instrument, as indeed we have done in Anchorage settings. A variation on the Troubleshooter for the Social Jungle (see pp. 80–82) for teenagers was developed for the training programs described below.

Training Program

Set out below is an outline of a 10 week group training program, with two 1½-hour sessions each week for a total of 20 sessions. This program is more intensive than most of the programs described in this book. Experience has shown that social skills acquisition cannot be hurried. For example, in a program described by Waksman (1984), 13 sessions of 45 minutes each produced changes in self-concept but not in assertiveness, for nondelinquent adolescents, compared with changes in a matched control group. The intensity and the procedures of Waksman's program are similar to others that have produced positive results, perhaps with a less ambitious curriculum. Thus, it seems that 10- to 15-hour programs are barely sufficient. In cases of severe skills deficits, such as typically encountered in delinquent teenagers, the intensity of training issue is even more critical.

The program described here is based on those developed in Anchorage under my consultation by David Glende of Alaska Youth Advocates for McLauglin Youth (detention) Center, and by Cheryl Gilligan for Booth Memorial Home (for youth detained for less serious offenses or attending day treatment on probation). It is modified to incorporate features of other reported programs, as acknowledged where applicable. It is assumed that the clients have been identified either as volunteers for social skills training in a detention facility or through some other screening process.

Session 1. Role play. The youths are given instruction and practice in role play as they might receive in a theater workshop. This practice does not focus on particular social situations, but provides basic skills for participation in later sessions. It is done before any role-play assessments are made, to help counteract the possibility that post-intervention evaluations may reflect acting ability rather than acquisition of social skills.

Sessions 2 and 3. Assessments. A full week is needed to administer pre-test evaluations for the dual purpose of modifying program content and contributing to an overall outcome measure. Assessments include questionnaires (e.g., modification for teenagers of Troubleshooter for the Social Jungle, see pp. 80–82), and role plays. Each client is videotaped in six separate social situations (standardized, following Michelson & Wood, 1982 and Goldstein et al., 1980). Although the accuracy of role plays for social skills assessment has been challenged (Kazdin, Esveldt-Dawson, & Matson, 1983), it does provide an opportunity for the trainers to see their clients in training-relevant situations.

Session 4. Introduction. Explanations of vocabulary such as assertive vs. aggressive vs. passive, suggested in most programs, are not necessary. We have found it more valuable to talk about "options" in the context of situations relevant to the group. For example: Your kid brother has borrowed your Walkman again and you can't find it; you have some options: lose your cool and hit him; express your frustration constructively; get a repayment by his delivering a card to your girlfriend's house. Thus, the purpose of the program is explained in terms of helping to develop options. We do not suggest taking away existing options, but to broaden the repertoire so that the teenager who chooses violence, drugs, or theft does not feel there was no other choice.

Session 5. Nonverbal communication. The appropriateness and the power of basic nonverbal expression is explored: mutual gaze, posture, qualities of voice, and others as listed at the end of Chapter 1. In this and the next two sessions, issues are raised in the context of generally relevant situations, and all group members participate in exploring them.

Session 6. Verbal communication. Particular emphasis is given to the impact of "I-messages," "you-messages," and feeling talk. Attention is also given to interpretive and listening skills.

Session 7. Emotions. Basic skills from the last two sessions are reviewed in the context of expressing and recognizing emotions. The essential suggestion is that if strong emotions are bottled up or, in the other extreme, vented indiscriminately, damage ensues. A working analogy that generally appeals is provided by the characters from Star Trek. Spock is ultralogical, McCoy is ruled by emotions, and Kirk combines rationality with his feelings; most youths aspire to emulate Captain Kirk.

Sessions 8 through 18. These sessions follow the format described in "Group Training Components" in Chapter 2 (p. 34): review; new topic; solutions; practice; feedback; feedforward; assignments. The practice (with role play), feedback, feedforward sequence is repeated as often as possible with different participants throughout the session. Each situation is analyzed in terms of six basic steps. Some elements can be expanded into subcomponents, depending on the sophistication of the clients. These six basic steps are:

- question
- respond
- predict
- suggest
- decide
- act

The steps are illustrated in the following sessions.

Session 8. Giving positive feedback. For example, recognition of how a classmate played in the basketball game against the staff.

Question: What was it you really liked?
Respond: "I really liked. . . . "
Predict: How will the other person respond to this compliment?
Suggest: If compliment rejected, reaffirm *other's* contribution; if receptive, restate *own* positive opinion.
Decide: "That's what I think."
Act: Smile, nod, shake hand, or other nonverbal closure.

Session 9. Giving negative feedback. For example, discovering a friend's failure to follow through on a promise.

Question: Can what you say really change things, or is it just a gripe? If negative feedback cannot be corrective, skip it.
Respond: "When you do . . . I feel. . . . "

Predict: Will the other person be threatened or will he or she care
about how I (or others) feel?
Suggest: "How about if you. . . . "
Decide: "I would be prepared to. . . . "
Act: "If you . . . then I. . . . "

Juveniles in institutions particularly enjoy this session, because they
discover that they can affect their own environment, including supervising staff, quite quickly.

Session 10. Accepting negative feedback. For example, reacting to
a supervisor who challenges a "shabby attitude."

Question: "Can you clarify. . . . "
Respond (reflective listening): "It seems that when I (do . . .) you
(react . . .)."
Predict: If you change in line with the complaint, how will that af-
fect you and the other person?
Suggest: Propose a change in your future behavior, do not worry
about the past. Suggest also how the other person might meet this
change.
Decide: "I would be prepared to. . . . "
Act: "If I . . . then would you. . . . "

Session 11. Making a request.

Question: What do you want and who should you ask?
Respond: Rehearse your wish: maximal clarity, minimum inconven-
ience. For example, "Can I look at that gadget for a few minutes
when you're through?"
Predict: Does this request really produce an imposition, or just a
standard moan?
Suggest: "We could trade. . . . " or "I've been waiting. . . . "
Decide: The request is worth asking, even if it is turned down.
Act: Make positive eye contact, smile, and ask.

Session 12. Apologizing. For example, feeling badly about a goof.

Question: Would you feel better if you talked about feeling bad?
Respond: Think about your own feelings, and express them to yourself.
Predict: How does the other person feel? When and where should we
bring the matter up?

Suggest: "Such-and-such has made me feel bad – perhaps you don't feel too hot about it either?"

Decide: Better to act quickly, not have it hanging. Speak out of caring, not out of guilt.

Act: "I feel . . . about . . . maybe you would. . . . "

Session 13. Dealing with peer pressure. For example, being invited to help disable an annoying supervisor's car or to share marijuana.

Question: Do you really want, for yourself, what is being suggested, or do you want to be part of the group?

Respond: "This is vandalism/assault/drug abuse. . . . "

Predict: "I'm on probation and if I'm caught that means two years. . . ; "

Decide: "Suppose we go down to Ch'cheezoo instead. . . . "

Act: Leave the situation: "If you can make it down there, I'll see you."

Session 14. Dealing with anger.

Question: Recognize the arousal: what is making you mad?

Respond: *Pause*, three large breaths; before speaking, take a bold and serious, but nonbelligerent, stance.

Predict: How to let off steam *and* feel better afterwards? Who is the best person to express myself to first?

Suggest: "I feel really irritated that. . . . "

Decide: "I have a right to my feelings, but there may be another side to the story."

Act: Express your point, listen actively, change the subject (both parties need to express themselves, feel that they have been listened to, but not necessarily resolved, if agree to differ).

Anger is important enough and difficult enough with some adolescents that an entire program can be oriented to the issue (e.g., see Feindler & Fremouw, 1983).

Session 15. Problem solving. For example, dealing with an annoyance.

Question: What is the problem and how does it affect you?

Respond: "When . . . (happens), I feel. . . . "

Predict: How can this situation change so that nobody loses?

Suggest: Propose several *different* alternatives.

Decide: Listen to the other opinions and agree on an alternative that can be done now.

Act: Start moving on the first step right away.

Session 16. Negotiating. For example, resolving a conflict of interest.

Question: What do *you* really want?
Respond: "I want . . . because. . . . "
Predict: What does the other person want?
Suggest: Propose a compromise or an exchange: "As a third option we could. . . . " or "What if we . . . this time, then . . . later?"
Decide: There are long-term, as well as short-term, benefits here, and the relationship is worth preserving.

Sessions 17 and 18. Specific issues. Two sessions are devoted to specific issues, identified earlier as relevant to some of the trainees. Development of strategies, guided by the six basic steps, is pursued.

Session 19 and 20. Assessments. Repeat the role plays and pencil-and-paper measures of Sessions 2 and 3.

There are many other skills that could be trained in further or alternative sessions (Goldstein et al., 1980, list 50 skills). One of particular value for girls concerns the response to unwanted sexual advances (in place of session 15 or 16). Those above are ones that we have identified as useful, interesting, and manageable in a 20-session course for teenagers. The teenagers worked with have most often been those apprehended, or identified as at risk for serious social problems. Thus many skills are necessary for their social survival, but their background and their resources most often leave them poorly equipped to develop these skills without direct intervention.

The six basic steps identified provide a "best fit" approximating structure to such a diverse group of skills – a very useful place to begin if not taken as a rigid formula. After brainstorming and experimenting within the group, it may prove satisfactory to supplement or reorder the steps proposed. Gilligan (see p. 176), in her applications of this program, has come to recognize the value of making it a task of the group to develop the steps for a given issue. It is helpful (sometimes necessary) for the trainer to have some previously determined task analysis to fall back on to provide hints and guidance without interference. This management of the group allows the trainees to develop a greater sense of control and self-efficacy.

For example, Gilligan's clients developed five steps for "expressing criticism" as follows:

1) Is it worth it?
2) Plan what to do (who to approach and how).

3) State the complaint (briefly, objectively).
4) Offer constructive alternatives.
5) Evaluate the outcome (with a view to continued improvement).

The interesting closure on this session was that another staff member happened by the group, and it was instantly decided that a real issue should be put to the test of these newfound strategies. A volunteer group member began with words to the effect of: "We've just been working on ways to express criticism . . . ." The exchange, watched with some intrigue by the group, came to such a satisfactory conclusion that it was spontaneously applauded. In a detention program for "predelinquent" behavior, effective ability to express criticism to authority has a high, natural motivation.

FAMILY CONCERNS

There are social skills training programs for adolescents of many descriptions other than "juvenile delinquents" (e.g., day-treatment programs for emotionally disturbed adolescents [Friedman, Quick, Mayo, & Palmer, 1983; Jackson, 1983] assertion training for middle-school students in health science classes [Waksman, 1984]). Nor is the institution the only setting for such programs.

It is impossible to leave this chapter without at least a brief mention of the extensive work by James Alexander and colleagues at the University of Utah. Although their work has been presented under titles of "systems-behavioral family intervention" and "behavioral family crisis programs," a notable focus has been on what they refer to as "destructive communication patterns." They have approached delinquency as a family communications problem – or, more exactly, they have approached delinquency as a problem in which family communications offers a solution.

In essence their approach has been to seek a curriculum indicated by family systems theory (see selected chapters in Gurman & Kniskern, 1981), following the methodology of behaviorism (cf. Stuart, 1980). For example, they target reciprocity and clarity of communication, using contingent reinforcement and discrimination training as major training strategies.

Many of the clientele were court-referred (for running away, trespassing, or minor drug offenses; see Alexander, Barton, Schiavo, & Parsons, 1976; Parsons & Alexander, 1973). Clear procedural information is provided in a book chapter by Alexander (1974). In this chapter he refers to defiant and coercive behavior in the family producing a balance of fluctuating forces – an uncomfortable but overall stable situation (the "homeostasis" of systems theory). The argument is that the delinquent behavior serves to hold the family together. For example, Alexander cites "Debbie," a teenager, who bickered with her mother and eventually started running away, with the result that her father stopped spending evenings "with the boys," returning home promptly from work in concern for his family.

The goal of family treatment programs following this rationale is to discover alternative ways to produce the required overall balance. One suggested means is a behavioral contract (see DeRisi & Butz, 1975). Contracts, more than anything, provide a forum for expressing opinions and desires. The process of training emphasizes:

- brevity
- directness
- personal responsibility for assertions or requests
- presentation of alternatives
- congruence (of verbal and nonverbal components) of messages
- concreteness (behavioral specificity)
- reflective listening

These emphases provide, in effect, a form of family social skills training not unlike those described in Chapter 6. The results are encouraging. Recidivism of delinquents in family treatment is consistently reported at or below the rate following other forms of intervention. Under optimum circumstances, in which therapist characteristics of structuring and relationship skills were maximal, Alexander and colleagues (1976) found *zero* recidivism in 12 months. These and other studies give considerable optimism to the prospect of putting together the puzzle of delinquency, in which social skill is a large and critical factor – yet only one of many pieces.

CHAPTER 11

Videotraining

The use of video considerably enhances one's scope in the training of personal skills. Two decades ago the videotape recorder and its accessories were being heralded as brave new technology ushering in a breakthrough for psychotherapy in general. That enthusiasm has been tempered for want of better empirical support, but it remains strong, and importantly, new optimism is in order following further technical developments and more informative research. Recording and editing devices have been improved and simplified, stimulated by the home video market. Research studies have recently started to address more precisely the interaction between tape content and individual personality. Overall, video offers a considerable expansion of capacity (more stimulation and greater variety of solutions), given a small investment of new expertise and a knowledge of potential pitfalls.

Video equipment is basically simple to use; some guidelines for further effectiveness in skills training are offered later in this chapter. Material in this chapter will also elaborate on the four major roles to be played by video in training programs for social skills. First, video provides a very convenient medium for presenting *scenarios* of problem situations to be addressed. These may include prerecorded tapes or role-played scenes of custom-made recordings. Second, prerecorded or specially created videotapes can provide modeled *solutions* to problematic situations. A third role for video is to provide *feedback* to the child who is struggling to master a new skill. Self-confrontation in this manner is useful in identifying skill deficits, if care is taken to preserve the person's self-esteem. However, it is probably more valuable to restructure the video replay, providing *"feedforward"* (the fourth role of video) rather than feedback. This terminology implies showing the child coping in a manner indicative of future performance not current performance. The use of moderately error-free video recordings is called *self-modeling*, probably the most powerful use of videotraining so far developed.

SCOPE OF APPLICATION

Before making a large-scale commitment to video technology in the cause of social survival it is advisable to make a sober survey of the general advantages and disadvantages that might accrue. If the commitment to social skills training is limited (e.g., till the grant runs out in November), then explorations in a new technology will be wasted. But otherwise, making an investment of time and effort will reap more and more benefits as the work proceeds with greater numbers of children over extended periods of time.

Advantages

Video can supplement and improve the functions of a social skills trainer in a number of respects. The first of these is an added dimension of *stimulation*. The television adds another medium; and changes between media, provided they do not overwhelm, are refreshing. Children will enjoy being passively engaged in different ways: watching and listening to the trainer or other children; reading words or drawings; watching or listening to recordings. Prerecorded material brings other people and other points of view into the room. Books, slides, and audiotapes can also achieve these purposes, but nothing else as readily available is as vivid as a moving picture. And children enjoy the technology. Growing up in a society in which television and the video arcade are major sources of recreation, and in which the educational plaything, the microcomputer, is hooked up to a video screen, today's children may almost expect to see a video recorder.

The second advantage is the possibility of *repetitive use* of some materials. Custom-made recordings are worth planning carefully, therefore. Or the recordings made spontaneously during training sessions may prove a valuable source of analysis. Some sequences may illustrate problems, progress, or mastery suitable for use in further training. (These should be edited into a usable format, catalogued, and safely stored [see Betts, 1983]).

When tapes produced over successive sessions are reviewed, they often indicate more progress than trainer or trainees remember – because with improvement the criteria for success surreptitiously increase. Such a review can be morale boosting and offer a basis for *evaluation*. To improve standardization, role-played situations can be predefined and videotaped at the beginning and end of training, later judged by trained raters according to specific criteria (see Maxwell & Pringle, 1983). Even if serious evaluations are not possible, simply an informal review of recordings will valuably assist a sense of direction for further training programs.

Another advantage of using video is the emergence of a wider *variety of solutions*. In reviewing prerecorded tapes, different people and perspectives are seen by the trainees. When video replay is used in the current session, trainees see themselves and each other in a different perspective. They also have the opportunity to examine the coping processes more thoroughly.

Finally, the increased availability of *home video recorders* brings a new possibility. Some tapes (or carefully selected extracts) may be beneficially reviewed further by the children involved. It is becoming more frequently possible to provide tapes for children to review at home, perhaps encouraging selected family and friends to view the tapes also.

Disadvantages

There are hazards in using video, both obvious and subtle. First, it involves some *expense* (to be discussed in more detail later), probably between $2,000 and $5,000 (in U.S.A., 1985), depending on the scope of the required system. However, funding agencies frequently will support equipment purchases. In any case, the total, multiple usefulness in the work setting needs to be predicted and evaluated against an appropriate time period. A less obvious, but maybe more important "expense" is the implied investment of expertise, the *time commitment* to mastering the equipment. The technical effort necessary is modest for the purposes of skills training, in contrast to that required for broadcast quality or art competitions. But further commitment to becoming acquainted with the psychological principles of application is necessary. These principles, not overly complex, are set out in the following pages.

One final word of caution. Any instrument that has the power to be effective has the power to harm. Video is no exception; there are *dangers* in its use.

If a solution to an interpersonal problem is inappropriately portrayed or misperceived by the observer, the persuasiveness of the medium can misdirect a viewer with harmful results. If a person is unprepared for the confrontation of their own self-image, and fallibilities are brought out insensitively, the emotional distress may reverse otherwise good progress. An understanding of the psychological dangers, described in appropriate sections throughout this chapter, has been clarified by research in recent years. In most cases, the pitfalls may be avoided by being alert and forewarned.

THE HARDWARE

Some readers will be fascinated by the intricate details of the technology; for them I recommend more extensive sources of information (e.g., Wallbott, 1983; Utz, 1980). Other readers may be dismayed by such details. But all video users will benefit from certain information, basic to choosing and operating the equipment. Readers who have access to technical assistance or who already use video equipment may well skip or skim this section.

Selection

Below is set out a *basic system*, assuming a wish to record, as well as replay, videotapes. If there are no initial plans to make recordings, the camera is clearly unnecessary but the remaining equipment should be selected with recording-compatible features. This strategy will greatly reduce the probability of kicking oneself later.

- video recorder: portable, including batteries, AC converter
- video monitor, 12"–19", color
- camera, hand-held, color, zoom lens, automatic focus
- videotapes (at least 10)
- cables

The advantage of the recorder being *portable* is simply one of flexibility. Even if training is based in a clinic or classroom setting, opportunities to record elsewhere often emerge. On the other hand, a nonportable type of recorder *may* facilitate editing. In place of a *monitor*, a regular television of reasonable quality may be used by way of an inexpensive accessory, an "RF converter," to the recorder. The screen size recommendations are determined by the need for it to be large enough to be seen by several people at once, compromised by the picture quality that occurs with larger screens. The advantage of a hand-held *camera* is again its flexibility; the zoom lens grants the ability to get close (providing detail) to a subject, and to vary the scope of the picture, without moving the camera. Automatic focus is advantageous for active clientele. *Videotapes* are reusable, but a budget for further supplies emerges from the frequent need to keep recordings. Expert guidance on the purchase of *cables* is necessary because there is a frustratingly wide variety of fittings and sockets in the video industry.

Useful *additions* to the basic system include (in some preferential order):

- microphone
- editing recorder
- editing console
- tripod
- lights

Portable cameras invariably have built-in *microphones*, often of high quality. However, these microphones are sensitive to all ambient noise, and are most receptive, inevitably, to noises close to the camera and those made by the camera itself. Thus, a separate microphone, close to and directed at the trainees, will enhance intelligibility of speech in otherwise distracting conditions.

The *editing recorder* provides a quantum leap forward in capability, in particular enabling the use of self-modeling. Crude editing (see later section on self-modeling, p. 201) can be achieved with any type of second recorder, and is often all that is required. Editing recorders are the most expensive item on the list (currently about $2,000 for reasonable quality) but they make operation much simpler, improve technical quality, and may enable such sophistications as recording backwards and fast or slow motion. The editing *console* enables smoother, more exact editing. It is not an expensive item in itself, but it will operate with recorders of specific characteristics only. Therefore, it is necessary to seek expert and trustworthy advice.

Hand-held cameras can be fitted to a *tripod*, stabilizing the picture as well as freeing the operator's hand. A regular camera tripod will do, given smooth swivel action, and easy height adjustment. Wheels (a dolly) are useful in only a few settings. Special *lights* are a low priority. It is probably better to spend more on a better camera that will operate under low-light conditions, and to look for unobtrusive ways to boost available illumination.

The *cost* of video equipment is remaining remarkably stable. Technological advances and growth of the home video market are bringing prices down at about the same rate as inflation is bringing them up. Functionally equivalent equipment costs the same dollar amount now as it did 10 years ago, and it is better quality, more robust, and easier to use. Expect to spend around $2,000 on the basic system; be very cautious about older equipment unless someone is giving it away. An editing system presently may cost twice as much as a basic system, but costs are coming down rapidly as the home video user has become a potential customer. The cost of tapes varies with type and quality. Budget $100 for tapes and at least an extra $100 for cables.

An important consideration not yet addressed is that of *compatibility* – largely a matter of tape format and recording speeds. The recording technology is complex and has undergone multiple revisions over the last 20 years without an industry standard emerging. (The situation was once similar for audio cassettes until Phillips gained sufficient control of the market to force other manufacturers to adopt their format.) At this time three *formats*, popular in the home video market, are worth considering for the price and quality appropriate to social skills training. These are VHS (Video Home System), Betamax, and 8 mm. Both VHS and Beta use half-inch cassette tapes, relatively light weight recorders, and a minimum of moving parts to produce quite high quality recordings. VHS is more widely used, but Beta technology apparently offers higher quality at lower cost. The 8 mm format is the newest and smallest. It has advantages that may eventually lead it to become the standard in the field. Already there are signs of Beta dropping out of the competition for home portable units. However, there are so many tapes available (mostly movies) in VHS and Beta that both these formats will be with us in table-top units for at least several years to come. A videotape recorded in one format is electronic gibberish in any other format, nor will it fit physically into a machine of another type.

Recorders and tapes that offer more than 2 hours (maximum) recording time under the current technology should be avoided. The length is achieved by slow recording speeds and thin tapes. Both attributes lead to a quality too poor to edit (editing involves rerecording, in which some of the picture "signal" on the tape is inevitably lost). As many as three different speeds are often available. Ideally, a system would record and edit at the fast speed, but be capable of copying and replaying at the other speeds. This ideal is seldom offered, so a compromise may have to be made.

The system primarily needs to be internally compatible. That is, tapes, recorders, and editors should be the same type. However, the monitor is not affected by format, and a camera has considerable versatility (seek a dealer's advice on the latter). Another consideration is compatibility with other video users. Two questions may be asked: Do you wish other people to be able to play your tapes? Do you wish to be able to play tapes produced by other people?

Operation

Video recorders are easily operated even by people who consider themselves nonmechanically oriented. The trainee operator should first watch how to use the equipment, practice under supervision, and have the manuals to refer to. Ultimately, the operator might teach someone else as the final step in the learning process. Here are some basic guidelines.

Because video is an electronic picture, its operation is a cross between a regular camera (e.g., 35 mm) and a cassette audiotape recorder. The *lens*, therefore, has variable aperture (f stops) and focus, qualities of depth of field. However, the recording is electronic, compensating to a limited extent for the amount of ambient light. Therefore, the picture will automatically brighten for a subject with a dark *background*, and darken with a bright background. Thus, the camera should be placed between the window and the subject; if this is not possible, it may pay to shade the window, even though the total illumination is reduced.

The *focus* is best adjusted with the lens zoomed in for maximum close up. The picture will then remain focused independent of the zoom unless the distance varies between camera and subject. The viewfinder is actually a miniature television-type screen, and shows exactly what is being recorded (though probably not in color). In most cameras this screen can be used for replay, to check recordings in the field. Early in the recording session it is important to verify the picture, and the sound using an earpiece.

The *monitor* should be disconnected during recording sessions. Otherwise, the audio causes feedback, and the picture distracts the trainees. Finally a note must be made of the *delicacy of the camera*. Very bright lights will damage the viewing screen in most cameras and create what appear to be holes in the recorded picture.

Troubleshooting

Below are some common *ailments* and their probable solutions. In all cases, check and recheck cables, plugs, power supply, and switch settings first.

During recording or first time playback

No picture
- check lens cap, camera cable, camera/VTR switch
- check power supply of recorder (and camera if separate)
- check brightness control on viewer/monitor
- try again and check that recording signal inside viewfinder is on

No sound
- a loose microphone cable will cut off the automatic without engaging the remote microphone
- if using a remote microphone, it may require a fresh battery

Faint picture
- check aperture setting
- insufficient light on subject
- check brightness controls

Unstable picture
- camera switched to "VTR"
- skew or tracking switch not on "auto"
- record heads need cleaning

Poor sound
- microphone too far away
- monitor left on during recording
- mismatched impedance between microphone and recorder
- radio waves or fluorescent lighting transmissions picked up by unshielded microphone cables

Recorder switches itself off
- batteries need recharging
- end of tape

Record function does not operate
- end of tape
- record protection holes on cassette not sealed

On replay of tape previously problem-free

No picture
- check VTR/TV settings on monitor
- check brightness control

No sound
- check channel 1/2/mix settings

Poor picture
- check brightness controls
- skew or tracking needs adjustment (probable if recording made on another machine)
- replay heads need cleaning

Poor color
- check hue and contrast controls

- color "temperatures" may have been on wrong setting during recording

Poor sound
- monitor malfunction

Replay function does not operate
- end of tape

SCENE-SETTING VIGNETTES

The simplest use of video in social skills training is to illustrate situations that promote discussion or problem solving amongst the clientele. The publishers' warehouses are not overly replete with products custommade for these purposes; nor does the scientific literature abound with descriptive and evaluative studies. However, a logical approach to examining the application of video vignettes will lead to the adaptation of existing materials or the creation of new ones.

Content

Recorded vignettes should be more than one minute, but less than five minutes long. To warrant setting up the equipment, the demonstration scenarios will need to be reasonably complex or subtle, in ways that cannot be readily conveyed without video. But scenes that are too long will appear either overly complicated or boring – an inefficient use of time.

The presentation is best made in the beginning (educational) phase of an individual session. The vignettes may present the current training topic in one of two ways: skill-oriented or problem-oriented. For example, if it is planned to dwell on the implications of mutual gaze, the depicted scene should demand eye contact (e.g., being accused of cheating) as a skill of more than minor importance. However, at this point the scenarios should avoid demonstrating the skill required – the function of modeling, described in the next section. Rather, the scene is one in which the target skill would make a significant contribution to an effective response. As set out in Chapter 2, later sessions are likely to focus on complex problems that draw a number of skills together for their solution. Scene selection for these sessions are thus problem-oriented. For example, the topic may concern how to deal with bullies. It would then be appropriate to show perhaps two or three unresolved sequences of one child being taken advantage of by another.

One of the scenes in the above case may include an unjustified accusation, thus coinciding with the material used for a skill-oriented session. The session may then be guided in alternative ways to determine whether a narrow set of skills is explored or a diverse number are drawn together around some problematic theme. For example, the tape may be viewed, followed with a question such as, "What should Gwendoline do now?" With guidance and prompting the appropriate topic will emerge. This topic can then be pursued with demonstrations, role play, and feedback as previously described. Video of the future will be an interactive device, which will expand its role in presenting complex situations with multifarious possible solutions. In the meantime, video assists the trainer with many dimensions of flexibility in the use of a single set of materials.

Sources

There exists a small, slowly growing supply of *materials developed specifically* for the purpose of scene setting. One is a complete package called *Asset* (Hazel, Schumaker, Sherman, & Sheldon-Wildgen, 1981). This program offers video vignettes for a variety of situations (e.g., following instructions, making conversation). It has been thoroughly developed and includes modeled solutions and training manuals for 8 sessions. It is also very expensive—currently $1,400—and is limited to use with young adolescents. Another source recently available is the *Accepts* program (Walker, et al., 1983). The manual is available separately and the tapes are cheaper (about $400). The vignettes run scene setting and responses together, providing both positive and negative examples. It is designed for mildly or moderately handicapped children from kindergarten through grade 6.

Several other resources are suitable for *adaptation*. A few instruments available on audiotape or videotape exist for assessment of social skills. These may be suitable as training scenarios with a minimum of adaptation. For example, Arkowitz et al. (1975) offer a series of audiotaped scenes from hypothetical dating situations. Although developed for university students, the tapes may be helpful for teenagers. Patricia Jakubowski (Jakubowski-Spector et al., 1973) produced over 20 vignettes on film, specifically to provoke an assertive (or other) response from the viewer. Once again, these materials were developed for adults.

There are compensations for the relative lack of child-oriented materials. Two considerations are of greater importance than the age of the actors: scene content and intelligibility. Much of the adult social world (courtship, employment) is less meaningful to children or may be portrayed too subtly (complex language, abstract referrents). But many themes are relevant at all stages of life: meeting strangers, dealing with authority, facing (or expressing) disapproval of loved ones, to list a few. Michael Mahoney's videotapes on provocation and anger control (Goodwin & Mahoney, 1975), for example, offer themes that are relevant to many ages.

If these themes are clear to children, it does not matter whether the actors are adults, puppets, or cartoons. Therefore, the imagination may be exercised in capturing suitable scenarios. The perfect vignette may already exist on a videotape of Pinnochio or Miss Piggy. Children respond very well to puppets, animals, and some fairy-tale characters because it puts the children in a nurturing position. The "lesser creatures" often promote more engagement, emotionally and intellectually, for otherwise unreceptive children. Children who are beyond this stage and provide good working rapport may find some benefit to their developing processes by responding to adults in a thematically relevant situation.

Finally, vignettes may be *created* by the children themselves, offering some advantages and some disadvantages. The biggest advantage in creating one's own materials is ensuring their relevance. Some children will get an ego boost from their ministardom, and will enjoy seeing themselves and each other. On the debit side, quality may suffer, not all children will enjoy the process, and for others the emotional interest will distract from the message. It may pay off to engage some acting students or to produce vignettes as a by-product to the uses of video described in later sections. It is often better if the actors do not play the part of themselves, but rather someone they know. In a bully scene, for example, Gwendoline, who is normally pushed around, plays the bully while another child plays Gwendoline. Such role reversals are often therapeutic in themselves and result in better acting by amateurs.

Developing vignettes will take time. They will require separate sessions devoted to the enterprise, additional to the established course of social skills training. The payoff will come later.

MODELING ON VIDEOTAPE

Following the scenario or situation definition, the discussion, and the other contributions of the trainees, videotaped model solutions are valuable. In one respect they may confirm solutions already proposed or practiced, thus boosting the sense of self-efficacy. Alternatively, the videotape may provide new solutions. In the commercially available recordings mentioned above, it will be necessary simply to stop the tape after a provocation scene to allow for input from the children, and then to continue the tape to demonstrate a suitable response. It is typical for modeling tapes and films to show both the context and the appropriate social skills. (For modeling purposes, videotapes and 16 mm films will be discussed as equivalent.)

Enhancements

Much more material is available and more descriptive research has been published in the area of modeling than in scene setting. Most often the modeling in social skills training is "live," but a large number of studies in other areas (e.g., treatment of phobias) exist to show that filmed models are only marginally less effective than live models (see Bandura, 1986). Other factors are generally more important. (General principles of modeling are reviewed briefly in Chapter 2, and in more detail in Chapter 3).

The more important factors include the perceived similarity between observer and model, and the coping nature of the modeled behavior. The study by O'Connor (1969) described in Chapter 3 provides a good example of a modeling film in which the actors were children of *similar* age to the clientele. However, more important than physical looks and age are behavioral similarities. Therefore, the choice of material may be determined by the social situation being portrayed and the individual's background skills to respond in that context: "Will these kids be able to relate to that?" The type of situation that is evocative of the skills demanded, and the abilities already evident will be the overriding considerations. Of additional importance will be characteristics of age, gender, race, education, and social and economic background.

The second major factor mentioned above is the value of a model seen to be *coping* rather than showing instant mastery of a situation. A flawed performance gives credibility, gradual solution to a problem offers considerable skills information, and final success provides hope and motivation. Other attributes to look for in a model are attractiveness and prestige, provided that these qualities do not distract from the coping nature of the model.

One Step at a Time

There are a number of ways to enhance the modeling process. There are universal advantages in analyzing skills into manageable components, ensuring that one is thoroughly mastered before proceeding to the next. Social skills are complex enough sets of behaviors that model tape or film materials should be carefully scrutinized before use. It may be necessary to omit sequences that do not meet the goals of the session.

Subdivision of the Recording

Stopping the tape or film at carefully selected points throughout can have several valuable effects. First, it may help to provide a finer task analysis. Also, it may be considerate to the attention span of the children in the training program. The ability to attend is highly variable across age and between individuals. Learning stops long before attention loss is indicated by a breakdown of self-discipline. Therefore, segments no longer than a few minutes long are recommended for any age group.

Stopping the tape allows for an approximation of "participant modeling" – the most powerful form of observational learning. That is, the observing children are given a chance to practice what they have seen while it is fresh in their memories. Neither the new set of skills nor remembering them should be too demanding. Thus, the probability of success is increased by using short sequences, and the whole experience is more naturally rewarding.

Subtitles

Further enhancements may derive from the addition to the recordings of a few clarifying words. The goal is to promote adaptive thought-action connections more directly. The cognitive-behavior therapists have shown that some self-talk can help to sustain a person through difficult situations, particularly when anxiety or anger are factors (see Chapter 5; Meichenbaum, 1977). Visible subtitles of key words will not distract from the action and will clarify the covert processes. For example, if the model is using cue-controlled relaxation, the best way to convey the exact timing is by the cue word showing on the screen. The key steps in Meichenbaum's self-talk approach can be used similarly.

If a more extensive commentary is desired, visual subtitles are not appropriate. However, *audio dubbing* can be used effectively. This technique has the advantage that it can probably be done without additional equipment. Most recorders have two audio channels, but the sound track needs only one. First ensure that a new recording can be made safely on one channel without losing the previously recorded sound. Additional commentary can then be dubbed onto the second channel following manufacturer's instructions for the video recorder.

Repetitive Presentations

Unlike live demonstrations, recorded models can be replayed numerous times before they wear out. The advantage for the trainee is that repetitive viewing allows more details of the task to be observed. On first viewing, there are limitations to what can be absorbed from a complex stimulus. Some aspects will be distracting to the intended purpose; for example, the funny shape of a person's ears, the color of the room. When the trainer encourages ignoring them, these aspects will quickly become habituated to. The global features of a skill will be all that can be appreciated on first viewing – and may be sufficient in some cases. But a practice run may indicate the need for better timing, more exact appreciation of content, or other nuances. These subtleties will be readily evident on repetitive exposure. Because the replications are exact, those aspects that have been absorbed on the first or second viewing are readily ignored in favor of different detail.

SELF-CONFRONTATION: VIDEO FEEDBACK

The trainer has set the scene, offered some demonstrations of how to deal with it, and encouraged the clientele to try out responses according to their own style; the trainees may then want to see how they are progressing. And the trainer may want to show them. I say "may" because video self-confrontation can be as dangerous as it can be effective.

The general purpose of showing clients themselves on videotape is frequently described as "feedback," as if that were an explanation in itself. Feedback has been established as valuable, and sometimes essential, to the process of learning specific motor skills. For example, it is impossible to ride a bicycle without kinesthetic feedback from muscles and balance organs. Research (e.g., Carrol & Bandura, 1982) is progressively clarifying the role of visual monitoring in the acquisition of new motor skills. However, social skills are quite a different matter, because of one critical circumstance: The skill definition and purpose are vastly more diffuse to the trainee.

Video replay does, of course, provide feedback in the sense that it offers a sample of data on previous performance. To make it useful, therefore, we have to narrow the definition of what is being learned to reduce ambiguity of the feedback for the client. Examples of positive benefits will be given later in this section, but first it is necessary to put aside some popular misconceptions about self-confrontation. Overall, it appears that video feedback has real but selected benefits, and should be used with caution.

Warnings

There has been much uncritical enthusiasm for the procedure of showing therapy clients their video image, as if simple video replay had inherent therapeutic benefits. Surveys of the research literature over the years have consistently concluded otherwise (Danet, 1968; Griffiths, 1974; Hung & Rosenthal, 1981). In most cases the results for the clientele are equivocal, in some they are detrimental.

The simple, but still commonly overlooked, fact is that viewing oneself on video has an emotional impact aside from its informational value. Some of this impact is simply arousal, which is transitory; therefore, reviewing a tape more than once may increase receptivity to the information component. But negative information (lack of skills, unsatisfactory outcomes) contributes to a loss of self-esteem. In a famous example, Schaefer, Sobell, and Mills (1971) found alcoholics more likely to drink after seeing their own drunken behavior on videotape. Even in less serious affronts to one's self-esteem, feedback of failure is bound to undermine one's sense of self-efficacy. Therefore, video replay to show errors can be undertaken only when it is considered to outweigh these disadvantages. (A study comparing feedback of errors vs. replay of success is described later in "Self-modeling," p. 201.) Some positive uses of video feedback are listed below (cf. Hosford & Mills, 1983).

Self-monitoring

Examples of one general skill – the ability to monitor accurately one's own actions – are precise enough to benefit from feedback. For instance, a child may be asked to count how often he interrupts, or initiates new topics of conversation. If his monitoring does not appear to match some independent observations, video or audiotape feedback may be used, clearly identified for the purpose. Most of the following suggestions are, in a sense, varieties of self-monitoring training.

Interpersonal Process Recall

Kagan (1978) popularized a procedure designed to improve recognition of thoughts and feelings associated with particular actions. By asking a child to relate what she was thinking or feeling at the time of the original activity while she watches a replay, two objectives may be achieved. First, the interconnections between cognition, affect, and behavior are clarified. Second, the child may come to see for herself which behaviors (or thoughts guiding them) are adaptive and which are not.

Personal Scientist

Video may be used to encourage some experimentation. Sometimes a child needs to undertake a major hurdle in his repertoire, but is reluctant to do so, maybe stating quite adamantly that "it won't work." For example, he may be overly inhibited about visibly expressing his feelings. In these circumstances it pays to take an empirical approach. He might be asked to playact over flamboyance; his inhibitions will almost certainly prevent him from real exaggeration. The video replay then allows the child to make an individual decision, perhaps to alter a "personal construct." This use of video would have been approved by Kelly (1955) who claimed that each individual is a personal scientist with a set of hypotheses (constructs) about the world – hypotheses that need to be tested and revised for adaptive living. In most respects, it is more akin to feedforward (self-modeling, see p. 201), than feedback.

Documenting Progress

If video recordings have been made over several weeks, they can be judiciously used for morale boosting. When progress is gradual, which it usually is, clients tend to forget their original levels of frustration or inability. The memory of one's pre-intervention abilities suffers severe interference from recent activities – with the result that due appreciation of progress is lost. Under these circumstances it is advantageous to select a previous recording (as early in training as possible) and show it, immediately followed by a recent recording of the same trainee(s) providing maximum contrast. If the manner of presentation engenders an upbeat, festive atmosphere, the event can stimulate considerable motivation.

Displaying Consequences

When a person is involved in a social interaction, it is impossible sometimes to be fully aware of the range and details of the interaction. That is, even when certain consequences are recognized, it may not be understood which specific actions lead to those responses. Video replay can usually fill the gap. However, it is essential to exercise particular care when the consequences are negative. Seeing what makes another person smile is always valuable. Recognizing the causes of another's frown is valuable *only* if it leads to an appreciation of how a smile might be won next time; even so, motivation and self-efficacy are threatened.

Nonverbal Components

Sometimes it is valuable to focus only on visual factors, simply achieved by turning off the sound during replay. Reducing the complexity of the stimulus by 50% makes the feedback more effective. If the content of what is being said needs more attention, the opposite procedure is applicable: listen to the recording with the picture off, or use audiotape only.

Still Frame; Variable Speed

A particular pose, expression, or visible interaction (e.g., eye contact) can be captured and emphasized with the "pause" button. The still-frame feature is particularly valuable for rare moments of success that need to be reinforced. Some recorders and all editing machines have variable-speed features, usually both forwards and backwards. The advantage of a high-speed replay is to emphasize repetitive mannerisms. The effect is comic, which may or may not be useful. Slow motion can help the identification of specific movements and their components. This need not be comic with the sound off.

The above strategies that involve tampering with sound, picture, and movement controls constitute restructuring of the video replay. Structured video replay, especially through editing, appears to offer interventions more powerful than simple feedback. These processes add greatly to the complexity of using video, however. Thus, the beginnings of a conceptualization are presented here.

A THEORY OF VIDEO REPLAY

All information is edited. From FBI reports to books on social skills training, communications are selected and structured for presentation. The individual consumer further selects and imposes a structure on the information available. Video replay offers no exception. Therefore, it behooves the scientist to discover the impact of the structuring process, so that the consequences, some of them dangerous, are not left to chance.

The general impact of video confrontation that includes errors or other activity not considered adaptive or desirable is *to identify targets* of change. Therefore, video replay containing errors is appropriate to training therapy only if the areas for improvement are not recognized or are incompletely understood. Video replay, after this fashion, serves more for assessment than for intervention. It is also a source of motivation because it highlights the *extent* of the deficits. This information produces a variety of emotions in the person confronted: guilt, embarrassment, depression. Such sources of motivation are clearly potent but dangerous because of their unpredictability.

The reason for the emotional reactions to video confrontation, I suggest, are as follows. It seems logical to suppose that generally, people are more critical of the present than of the past or the future. There is survival value in being vigilant about one's current circumstances because of the opportunity to maneuver. Being observant of how I am coming across to my audience allows me to alter my style and improve the outcome. However, the past cannot be changed, so there is some survival value in a memory that emphasizes positive events, notwithstanding a minority of unforgettable horrors. (Clinically depressed people provide an exception to this generalization.) It would be functionally unbearable to live with family, colleagues, or friends if this selectivity were not so. Likewise, the future is anticipated rosily to make getting up in the morning possible, if not desirable.

Video replay brings the past into the present. The viewing takes place in the present, so our critical vigilance operates reflexively. But the action on the screen cannot be altered in response to this vigilance, causing the inevitable emotional reactions. For the video self-image to be responded to without emotional sabotage, it must present a positive-to-negative event ratio comparable to that provided by selective memories of the past or natural optimism of better things to come.

The process of self-modeling, described below, is both natural and logical, under the reasoning presented here. To suggest that clients should see unedited videotapes of themselves is like suggesting that scientific articles should go to press without a review process.

SELF-MODELING: VIDEO FEEDFORWARD

Self-modeling is the process in which video replay is structured to show only adaptive behaviors. The resultant tapes are normally kept brief (2 to 5 mintues) and shown repetitively (e.g., six times over 2 weeks). The technique pulls together elements of observational learning (in that is shows coping skills) and video self-confrontation (in that the subject observes himself or herself) in a way that enhances self-efficacy (by emphasizing success). In philosophy, it is a "feedforward" rather than a feedback technique, because it aims to give information about how the subject *might act in the future*, not how he or she has been acting in the recent past. The video recording is constructed *to define* the behavior adaptive of future functioning, at the same time avoiding the negative emotional reactions that inevitably result from reexperiencing immutable, past events. It is generally in the trainee's interests to talk of the self-model as descriptive of the future.

After a brief discussion of efficacy, this section will offer more details on the method of implementation and description of some specific examples. For reviews of self-modeling in a larger context than social skills training, see Dowrick (1983b) and Hosford (1980).

Efficacy

In its brief history, self-modeling has been shown to be effective in a variety of areas. Studies so far reported include targets of physical skills (e.g., swimming, Dowrick & Dove, 1980; powerlifting, Maile & Dowrick, 1985), vocational skills (e.g., teaching, Hosford & Polly, 1976; packing assembly, Dowrick & Hood, 1981), communication (e.g., assertiveness, Creer & Miklich, 1970; stuttering [audiotape], Hosford & Brown, 1975), and personal adjustment (e.g., hyperactivity, Davis, 1979; depression, Prince & Dowrick, 1984). More than half of the applications have been with children; in fact, examples can be found in self-modeling directly applicable to the topics of Chapters 3 through 9 of this book.

The variety of studies reported include many forms of analysis. There are case studies, some of which used reversal or multiple baseline designs. Others have used group designs with between-group or within-subject comparisons. In some instances, control conditions have offered credible placebos or simply no treatment. More recently, there have been comparisons with other active treatments such as token economies or video replay of errors. In all cases, self-modeling has been reported superior, despite the remarkable brevity of the intervention.

Perhaps most relevant in the present context is to describe a study comparing self-modeling with an "error-learning" procedure. The study provides an analogue only, for the target behavior was a variation on pool playing (chosen for its simplicity of study). The subjects were 18 evenly matched pairs of pool players who competed with each other twice. After the first round, losers only were assigned to either a self-modeling or an error-learning condition. Tapes were edited to show, in the first case, only successful (self-modeling) shots and, in the second case, only the missed shots (error-learning). Subjects then observed their edited tapes for 2 minutes on six occasions spread over approximately 2 weeks. After the rematch, it was simple to compare the subjects' performances both with their own earlier play and with that of their matched comparison subjects. In terms of the absolute number of successful shots, *all* subjects in the self-modeling group showed increases, whereas less than half the other players improved these scores. In terms of the absolute number of unsuccessful shots (which varies somewhat independently of success), *all* subjects in the error-learning group did worse relative to their opponents.

This study helps to clarify why unstructured video replay produces equivocal results. Other studies have supported the differential effects of replaying desired versus undesired behavior. For example, Kehle, Clark, Jensen, and Wampold (1986) used self-modeling with hyperactive children in the classroom, following a multiple baseline design. Three children viewing edited adaptive functioning improved while a fourth child watching unedited tapes became more disruptive (he subsequently reversed his behavioral trend on watching a self-model tape). It is also apparent, at least with adults, that those with lowest self-esteem benefit most from self-modeling (Germaine & Dowrick, 1985).

Unfortunately, a minority of the video literature is devoted to replay structured to emphasize adaptive solutions to future problems. Most practice remains oriented to uncensored replay for the purpose of insight analysis into past behavior.

Methods

There are several different approaches one can use to create a self-model recording for feedforward purposes. It is best to combine several of these approaches according to one's needs and resources. An overview of procedures to produce and implement the self-model recording is outlined in Table 11.1. (A demonstration film, Dowrick, 1978a, and training videotapes for different applications of self-modeling are also available.)

The original method used to create a self-model was simply to videotape a rehearsed *role play* of adaptive behavior. As described by Creer and Miklich (1970), this application involved a 10-year-old boy with conspicuous social skills deficits, who had failed to respond to either tradi-

TABLE 11.1
Elements of Creating a Self-model Videotape*

Maximize the child's performance *during* recording by:
   • incentives ("You can see yourself on TV later")
   • verbal encouragement
   • physical support (out of camera's view)
   • flattering camera angles
   • rehearsed role play
   • relaxation or medication to reduce anxiety or overactivity
   • patience
Collect sufficient recording (probably 10 to 20 minutes) to create a self-model.
Extract the best by *editing* to:
   • remove mistakes
   • repeat adaptive sequences
   • resequence events
   • delete evidence of support
   • enhance aesthetics
   • insert from other material
Complete a self-modeling tape of 2 to 5 minutes, depending on the age of the child and the complexity of behavior
Present the tape at regular, spaced intervals (e.g., six times over 2 weeks)
Monitor progress and repeat with new recordings as necessary, involving the trainee as much as possible
Combine with other intervention strategies

*Adapted from Dowrick, 1983b

tional psychotherapy or contingency management. In lieu of any other available modeling procedure, self-modeling was devised and found to be successful. The recording was achieved through a script in which the youngster reacted adaptively to threats of bullying by peers and to other situations. There are obvious limitations to the role-play procedure; these have been addressed by two other major approaches: camera work and editing, both made possible by recent technology.

Camera work refers to the ability of a mobile camera with a zoom lens to select (or even distort) specific elements of the environment. Thus, to show a girl what it looks like for her to stand up for herself, she can be filmed with her supportive big sister standing behind her – but out of the picture during recording. The fact that she remembers the presence of her sister in the past event is not as important as creating a picture that defines her potential behavior in the future. The zoom lens can also play optical tricks: the telephoto can shrink the apparent distance between people. This feature can be useful in treating shyness (see case study of Charles in Chapter 3, p. 51). The wide-angle lens can make people look smaller.

When the recording has been made to include as many instances as possible of the target behavior, *editing* can be done to enhance it further. Ideally, these manipulations are made using specialized editing equipment. Note that the technology of videotape absolutely prohibits cutting and splicing (except in dire emergencies of salvaging a physically damaged original). Editing is done electronically by rerecording. For the present purposes, much editing can be achieved by copying onto any other recorder connected with appropriate cables. By editing in this fashion, the screen will lose picture momentarily at most of the "joins." (These faults will become a source of annoyance and diminished efficacy only if discrete sequences are short and numerous.)

In the simplest case, it may be necessary only to remove errors. Following a careful review of the original tape, the sections that need to be deleted can be memorized or documented. The tape may then be simply copied onto a tape in another recorder using the pause control on the second machine to eliminate unwanted sequences. It is also easy to record multiple copies of events particularly worth emphasizing.

With sophistication, there are possibilities of more illusory effects. For example, an early event may make eminent sense as a demonstration of a possible consequence to a later event; or material may be included from other recordings altogether. It bears repeating here that authenticity is not an issue. Subjects watching these tapes are not concerned with what they "really did." This issue is illustrated by many examples in which the subject collaborates in devising the self-modeling material and in selecting the material to be edited. This practice is to be encouraged as both effective and more ethically desirable. It avoids the question of clinicians imposing their ideas on helpless others if a child can say: "There's the me I want to be – let's have a closer look at that."

The edited tape with suitable repetitions should end up being 2 to 5 minutes long. It can be reviewed up to six times, depending on boredom or resulting improvement of skill level – usually both occur together. It seems best for the reviewing sessions to be spaced with one or two days in between. Systematic research on these parameters is lacking, but experience continues to confirm the effective viewing times for self-modeling (e.g., see Maile & Dowrick, 1985). If clients can review tapes on their home video recorders, there exists a very cost-effective system. Telephone calls can be made at prearranged times as reminders to review the recording.

If no form of electronic editing is available or logistics prevent repetitive viewing, the principles of self-modeling can be incorporated *without editing* into an immediate replay situation for *in vivo self-modeling.* First, a recorded sequence should not be replayed at all if it is known to contain a high proportion of poor responses (or even a low number of positive instances of the targeted skills). Those segments that are replayed should be given as much structure as possible, following these suggestions:

- Avoid comment on mistakes, but give considerable praise to success.
- Make the praise meaningful by pointing out causal relationships between specific behavior of one person and the reaction of another.
- Fast-forward longer sequences that are known to contain few benefits.
- Still-frame particularly good examples.
- Model and encourage supportive remarks amongst all those reviewing the tapes.

In short, help the trainees to selectively perceive the interactions that will lead to adaptive future functioning.

Examples

Two sample cases will be briefly described here. They are chosen because they represent very different target behaviors, and also they demanded quite different levels of sophisitication in the approach.

Childhood aggression. In this case, a particularly athletic 3-year-old boy "Steve" was terrorizing the neighborhood (at least those up to 7 years old), and getting along very badly with his mother. The problem was recast as one of poor child-parent communication. Steve had to learn how to get what he wanted from his mother without tantrums, and she had to learn how to convey her appreciation of his (rare) examples of socially acceptable communication. Steve was so noncompliant that when he let up, his mother was too exhausted to respond positively, although she understood effective parenting principles and wished to apply them.

Mother and son attended a psychiatric unit of a general hospital. Video recordings were made of their interactions in a playroom. As the nature of the problem emerged, the mother was directed to interact in certain ways in connection with a cooperative play situation. Although adaptive responding by mother and son was too infrequent for the encounter to be deemed in any way happy, during a one-hour session it was possible to capture a reasonable number of positive interactions on videotape.

These interactions were edited onto two tapes. One showed predominantly successful target behavior on the part of the mother, the other showed the child being socially adaptive. (Making two recordings was not necessary in principle, but served a purpose in the scientific analysis of the study [see Dowrick, 1978b].) Both clients watched first one tape repetitively over several days, and then the other tape. Observations were made of their subsequent interactions in the playroom, with daily reports recorded by the parent at home.

The overall results after a few weeks of this treatment were highly positive, and the improvements by each individual correlated with the tape under review. In this case, the creation of self-models was achieved mostly by the straightforward procedure of bringing together low-frequency but naturally occurring events. Other contributions came from using a setting that provided maximum support, encouraging maximum participation (the presence of a camera and the incentive of "seeing yourself on TV" can be played to advantage), and occasionally editing together events that, in fact, had been separated by an undesirable occurrence.

Selective mutism. Deficits in social conversation occur as a result of either inability or skill inhibition. The latter can occur in children such that the inhibition is strongly situation-specific, termed *selective mutism* (Kratochwill, 1981; also see Chapter 9).

A slightly different application of self-modeling was used successfully with two children ("Wendy" and "Joshua"), who spoke freely in their homes but nowhere else – most notably not at school (Dowrick & Hood, 1978). Selective mutism is very difficult to treat and a variety of procedures had been attempted in the 6 to 12 months that the children had attended school. The intervention that eventually proved to be successful involved videotaping the children at home, using materials from school as a backdrop (e.g., alphabet charts). After making transcripts of those tapes, we arranged other recording sessions in the school to make it possible to edit together different sequences and produce a self-model that was essentially a Hollywood-style "fake." That is, material from one setting was interspersed with that from the other to make it look as if each child was answering questions and making comments at school. Cuts from one scene to another were very crude, so it was obvious what had been done. However, both children subsequently responded to reviewing their own tape (but not the other's) with improvements to a good level of adaptive classroom functioning.

The study provides an interesting example of a case in which self-modeling worked where peer modeling was ineffective. Both children were, of course, surrounded by classmates who spoke freely but were not responded to as models. After the self-model tapes had been constructed, both children watched one tape only: that is, Wendy saw her own tape while Joshua observed it too. This continued for a number of sessions (phase 1). The other self-model tape was then used (phase 2) so that both children watched Joshua's tape, and the procedure was repeated for two more phases. Effectively, over four phases, each child saw a self-model while the other observed a peer model. Systematic observations revealed that changes accrued during self-modeling only, and were maintained during peer modeling. The changes were also noted to be long lasting, as evidenced by formal observation after 6 months, and informal observations a year later.

CONCLUSION

The various approaches offered by videotape in this chapter can be used independently of one another. Alternatively, they fit together in a natural sequence as follows:

- Scenes are set with video *scenarios*.
- Trainees attempt their own *solutions*.
- Videotape *models* are reviewed.
- Video recordings are made while trainees *practice* revised skills.
- These recordings are reviewed to provide constructive *feedback* on current performance.
- Trainees *refine* their role-played skills for the camera.
- Structured versions of the recordings offer *feedforward* via self-modeling.
- Trainees *perfect* their skills in role play, with assignments, and in real situations.

As the horizons expand with increased knowledge, more research, rather than less, is called for. This research will refine the knowledge of video procedures. We will gain sophistication in scenario presentation to make more accurate impact; our knowledge of appropriate characteristics of models will improve their relevance for children of different backgrounds. More ways will be found to structure video replay and to vary the length, frequency, and complexity of effective sequences. But in the meantime, there is much to work with. We now know enough to be able to operate, with effectiveness and safety, an instrument of considerable power.

CHAPTER 12

Professionals in Child Help

Professional concern for children and their social survival gives rise to some very special considerations. Children are *dependent*, in varying degrees, both practically and legally. Thus, people in professional roles must frequently make judgements with greater responsibility and less client contribution than when working with adults. Furthermore, direct intervention with social skills is a recent but rapidly spreading strategy that lacks established boundaries. The scope of training and the professions with responsibility, or even permission, to offer it are topics now reaching the public forum. This chapter presents some beginning considerations.

PROFESSIONAL ROLES

Three major issues arise from considering who should do what to whom, when the "what" are training social skills and the "whom" are children. These issues revolve around family responsibilities, boundaries between professions, and individual limits to intervention. The major theme in defining social skills, as presented in Chapter 1 and echoed throughout this book, is that of learnable units of behavior that enable a child to become more versatile in social situations.

Professions or Parents

The maximum involvement by parents in training programs is desirable both for improved efficacy of training and for ethical reasons. However, the question may be raised of whether social interaction styles are too personal for professional intervention except in extreme cases. Social skills may be seen to overlap with manners, morals, and conventions best determined by family value systems, giving rise to a debate on similar principles to that which surrounds sex education in school. Some critics have claimed that assertiveness and social skills taught in schools have dulled the individuality of children (see discussion by Timnick, 1982). In this debate, the opinions range from the absolute extremes of giving total responsibility to the family or carte blanche to the schools, but most often center around where to draw the lines of responsibility.

To resolve these differences of opinion, the channels of communication must be kept open. Some parents, unfortunately, will not care. Others, however, will be concerned that training of social behavior is not appropriate unless the child is manifestly at risk and beyond parental guidance. Yet others may perceive a combat setting in which the professional and child are collaborating to compete with the parents.

A strong case can be made for teaching social skills as part of the regular classroom curriculum. The case has been made on the basis of better academic fulfillment (Cartledge & Milburn, 1978) and prognosis for mental health (Frosh, 1983). Some school districts in the United States have mandated at least a few credits of "life skills" into their programs and other districts are presently considering doing so. Such programs will face the parental challenges mentioned above, and the need to justify the objectives and content of training. Some researchers have criticized the current methods in social survival for children for insensitivity to individual variations in the development of friendships and other liaisons (Putallez & Gottman, 1983).

Parents need, first, to be informed. Second, they need to be reassured that the instruction is relatively free of teacher-imposed values. An emphasis that social skills provide *choice* is essential to this reassurance. However, options made possible by a teacher will often carry an implied positive value or preference. Therefore, teachers should welcome the involvement of parents, so that the school-provided educational opportunities supplement rather than compete with family ideals.

Demarkation Disputes

The professions of childcare are not demarked, fortunately, by the rigid boundaries that in some of the labor force set truck drivers idle all day because they are forbidden to unload their own vehicles. However, boundaries do exist, often vague, seldom legally explicit, sometimes sources of bitterness and conflict. I have written this book in the hope of it being interesting and useful to a wide range of professions: program coordinators, clinical psychologists, classroom teachers, special teachers, occupational therapists, social workers, psychiatric nurses, pediatricians, psychiatrists, childcare workers, and many others, whether they primarily study, research, or practice in these and related areas. Each person must function according to the scope of his or her profession.

It is not, I think, a question of "which profession is responsible for the social survival of children?" It is simply that each person may practice what she or he is trained to practice, within legal and ethical bounds. All personnel in the child-helping professions can contribute to the social survival and enhancement of children in their care, through direct services or by recognizing an appropriate course of action and recommending another source of help. In university courses that I have conducted on social skills training with children, education students frequently debate the respective territories of regular and special classrooms. Eventually, they agree that both have a role in the social survival of children. The debate shifts to a recognition of differences, according to professional training, in curriculum and populations. Thus, the distinction between these and other professions lies in recognizing what is to be trained, which children to work with, and identifying the limits of one's own resources so that appropriate referrals can be made.

Limitations: Referring Children On

"First do no harm" is a principle important not just to the medical profession, but to all human services. Fundamental to the application of this principle is the ability to recognize what can be done and the willingness to acknowledge when someone else is better placed to do it. These abilities depend on *information* (the purpose of this book), *self-appraisal*, and *perceptiveness*. For example, an individual childcare worker may have the expertise to train skills of, say, expressiveness, be able to recognize those as deficits in a particular child, but need the additional perceptiveness to recognize that this child may find some extraneous payoff for failing socially. The program is then limited by a type of sabotage that needs to be addressed with more intensive clinical resources. Listed below are some basic guidelines for circumstances appropriate to referral for more intensive therapy than is usually provided in group social skills training. Professional pride may seem to stand in the way of referral; rather, a professional pride "countercondition" should be developed with respect to the ability to identify effective referrals in the child's best interests.

Lack of progress. All children should make at least minimal, identifiable progress with little delay. Social skills, as described in this book and other programs referred to, are "learnable." Thus, lack of progress indicates inappropriate assessment or intervention. If the assessment and intervention strategies have been conscientiously devised, the existence of a more complicated condition of the child is implied.

Personality clash. The term is perhaps overly dramatic, but no trainer can be all things to all trainees. A program offers poor prognosis for reluctant clients. Enthusiasm is frequently generated by the trainer, but individual differences make it unrealistic to expect 100% rapport. Arnold Lazarus (1981), one of the world's most sought after clinical psychologists, makes a point of advocating quick referrals in circumstances of therapeutic-style mismatch; he actually *asks* clients what they look for in a therapist (e.g., sergeant major with a heart of gold). Working with socially deficit children, however, demands that the trainer attempts to recognize and be realistic about differences in style.

Bizarre behavior. Even socially unskilled children should be reasonably predictable. Behavior judged inappropriate but coherent with the referring condition of the child is most likely the expected target of the training program. However, if the behavior seems "bizarre," then the program is probably not designed to cater for it, and another opinion should be sought.

Disruptive behavior. An individual judgement is called for when disruption occurs in a group. If the program is for aggressively delinquent teenagers, then trainers will expect to manage more disruptions than if the program is for socially isolated preschoolers. However, all groups have their limits of tolerance. The basic guide is the consideration to all members of the group. The decision to retain or refer a disruptive participant should reflect the best interests of him or her and other participants.

Emerging problems. Whereas screening may have been carried out in the best of faith, sometimes children will reveal complicating problems after training has begun. Medical or emotional problems should be referred immediately. Evidence of abuse must be reported (see "Legalities and Ethics," p. 219)

Unwillingness. Clients of human services always have the right to withdraw (also an ethical issue). Because children are dependent—more so those with social deficits—it is incumbent on trainers to be alert for change of heart in their youthful clients. A confused or depressed child may respond to reassurances, or may need a diplomatic opening to discontinue before more damage than good is achieved.

CHANGING SOCIAL BEHAVIOR

The techniques for change described in this book are ones that, primarily, have developed out of a behavioral approach to psychology. The advocated trainer style, and much of the curriculum content, is imbued with humanistic methods and values. Overall, these behavioral-humanistic techniques are characterized as *directly* addressing social deficits. The major categories of *indirect* intervention, psychotherapy and drug therapy, are summarized here to provide a contrast.

First, however, the behavioral-humanistic approach deserves some clarification. My conceptualization of behavior therapy, as characterized by its empiricism, is not without good company among recent formulations (cf. Kazdin, 1978, pp. 373–383; Marks, 1982; Wilson, 1978), but it strays somewhat from earlier definitions that insisted on a basis of learning theory (e.g., Wolpe, 1969, 1983).

Characteristics of Behavior Therapy

I characterize behavior therapy with the following seven features:

1) Assumption: there exists a behavior that may be changed to the person's benefit. This assumption does not imply, necessarily, that behavior must be observable, nor that behavior change is the only path of benefit.

2) Philosophy of approach: intervention begins at the most amenable point. This philosophy implies that observable is better than nonobservable, that current is better than past. However, it does not preclude unearthing the most distant associations or dealing with the most complex or intangible behavior (e.g., intuitions, dreams), should more direct approaches fail; it merely suggests a hierarchy of approach.

3) Specificity: targets of change, their circumstances, their impact, and associated concurrent events are described in unambiguous terms.

4) Measurement: assessment in terms of frequency, duration, and intensity allows determination of intervention recommendations and evaluation. Targets specified under 3) are measured to verify understanding of the problems and credibility of intervention.

5) Intervention: a technique is selected – identified as the most likely to succeed in bringing about desired change within a specified period of time. The client's collaboration in goal setting and choice of intervention is maximally sought. Most frequently in behavior therapy, the intervention has a learning theory rationale (e.g., operant conditioning). However, sometimes it does not. Not infrequently, a technique is developed with a theoretical rationale that is later disputed, even though the efficacy is not (e.g., systematic desensitization was originally proposed as a process of reciprocal inhibition, but it is now arguable that desensitization occurs for quite different reasons; see Chapter 4; Kazdin & Wilcoxon, 1976; likewise, I believe self-modeling needs a different explanatory mechanism from that which prompted its development; see Chapter 11).

6) Monitoring: relevant behavior and related events are continually and closely monitored, allowing frequent modifications of intervention.

7) Review: goals for intervention are evaluated at predetermined time intervals. The purpose of these reviews is to judge if the behavior change as planned has occurred *and* if the behavioral changes have brought about the benefits originally desired by the clientele. Reviews are used to change goals, revise intervention choices, advise re-referral, or terminate therapy.

Characteristics 3 through 7 may be seen as procedural steps that may be repeated. Multiple targets and/or multiple intervention strategies are often engaged concurrently. The first two characteristics can be neither proved nor disproved; they represent acts of faith, like axioms to a scientific system. Thus, behavior therapy cannot be found right or wrong, but it can be found useful or useless. Pragmatically, there is mounting empirical evidence that the behavioral-humanistic approach to social skills training reported in this book is successful. Should some other approach prove more useful, then the basic acts of faith may be discarded or revised.

The net effect of the behavioral approach in contrast to others is an emphasis in therapy on *solutions rather than causes*. This emphasis appears to make behavior therapy more effective than popular. Research in chronic depression indicates that people with this disorder are characterized, above all else, by a tendency in the face of unpleasantness to ask, "Why did this happen?" as opposed to, "What can I do about it?" Since solutions are characteristic of people free of psychological disorders, therapies emphasizing solutions are bound to be more successful. They are bound, also, to be less popular, since people seeking therapy will be seeking causes. (See Dowrick, 1986, for a more extensive argument along these lines.)

Psychotherapy

Another set of assumptions underlies techniques fitting loosely under the umbrella of "psychotherapy" (see George & Cristiani, 1981). Whereas these two major systems are not necessarily incompatible, they lead to fundamentally divergent approaches. The basic assumption (listed as 1) above) of behavior therapy is not disputed, but it is simply irrelevant to psychotherapy. The assumption here is essentially that observable problems (e.g., aggressiveness, withdrawal) are the manifestations of inner conflicts. Many other characteristics of the approach are consequently different from the preceding list: interventions *begin* by probing beneath the surface; the manifestation of therapeutic change is to be discovered, not predicted, and therefore, goals cannot be set as they are for behavior therapy. That is, a psychotherapist will plan the intervention process and let the outcome emerge; a behavior therapist will plan a therapeutic outcome and set about discovering the intervention.

Overall, the result of a psychotherapy orientation to social skills is to proceed indirectly. Play therapy, for example, is designed to encourage the expression of conflicts, through fantasy, which the child cannot articulate. Dream interpretation explores symbols of desires and anxieties that are repressed by the conscious mind. It is proposed that bringing these conflicting needs and fears into consciousness will allow normal development to occur. Furthermore, it is often claimed that removing the "symptoms" (e.g., aggression, withdrawal) without addressing the underlying conflicts will result in temporary relief, followed by the emergence of new problems. However, the evidence for symptom substitution is sparse (according to behaviorists [see, Kazdin, 1978], removal of problem behaviors results more often in adaptive generalizations than in the emergence of new problems).

Drug Therapy

In the heyday of psychotropic medication prescriptions, 200,000 children in the United States were being given amphetamines for hyperactivity; in the vast majority of cases academic and social functions were not monitored (O'Leary, 1980). These drugs have since been shown to have side effects (e.g., stunting physical growth), and to have been overprescribed, in terms of both dosage and diagnosis. Drugs for other social disorders have followed similar, but numerically less significant, trends.

Notwithstanding the dangers and the criticisms, medications can be dramatically successful in properly diagnosed cases (see Werry, 1978). The fundamental assumption here, obviously, is that organic deficits can result in specific social dysfunctions. These organic deficits are thought to be functional, rather than structural, with a resulting imbalance of neurotransmitters in the brain. If this assumption is true, then it is logical to seek chemicals that can affect the central nervous system, if such drugs can be found that are reasonably specific to the chemical imbalance of the brain. Or drugs may be found that alter the child's receptivity to other therapies. Different environments, behaviors, and emotional states will also alter the brain, at least to some degree (see Kalat, 1984).

Oddly, psychiatric medicine has proceeded with less logic than has psychology. Psychotropic medications have been discovered by chance as often as predicted by chemistry. Ritalin (methylphenidate), the most commonly prescribed medication for hyperactivity, is an example. No one would have used a stimulant to tame activity if it had not been fortuitously observed. For years a controversy raged over these apparently "paradoxical" effects. The logical, though still not universally accepted, answer is that hyperactive children are underaroused, like cranky kids who should be in bed (Zentall, 1977).

Thus, it seems that drug therapies are generally applied as treatments of the behavior, but are officially defended as remedies for the underlying cause. In any case, both psychotherapy and drug therapy, as with the behavioral approach, have axioms, which may not be falsifiable in the scientific sense. Their acceptance depends ultimately, not on logic, but on empiricism: What is most effective? This question has an answer that must be continually revised.

JUDGING EFFECTIVENESS

Gradually, as the science of psychology matures, some procedures are emerging (for some conditions, or some populations) as more effective than others. It may sound astonishing to say so, but 10 or 20 years ago this was arguably not the case. That is, several approaches may be equally effective, for example, in treating bed-wetting or social anxieties. Therefore, professionals were justified in following an orientation in which they had been trained, and using a narrow range of techniques with which they were most familiar. Now, however, it has become increasingly important to evaluate a case on its merits and apply those techniques with *demonstrable* efficacy. The day is approaching when psychologists will be both legally and ethically accountable for their choice of interventions, as well as the expertise with which they apply them (cf. Risley, 1975).

In the context of social skills training, all procedures described in this book must be examined critically for demonstrations of efficacy. Some procedures have well-established track records; others with sketchy support are cited for lack of competition. In all cases, the evidence continues to trickle in, and it is necessary for us all to stay abreast of the evidence and to examine it critically with a view to revising our methods of intervention. Here are some guidelines (see Campbell & Stanley, 1966; Johnston & Pennypacker, 1980 for detailed discussions of evaluating applied research):

- Case studies are valuable only for unusual conditions or for descriptive details of new procedures. Multiple clinical cases are more valuable, provided assessment and client selection processes are clear.

- Single-case experimental and multiple baseline designs are informative of specific procedural elements and their impact on specific individuals. They include scientific controls not present in clinical case studies, but the results must be generalized with caution.
- Group studies allow more generalization of results, but obscure the importance of individual differences.
- Group comparison studies of procedures are frequently touted as ultimately the most valuable. However, a critical examination of methods must be made to equate procedures: in what sense are the comparative techniques "given an equal chance"? Technique A may surpass technique B because the practitioner is much better at A or took more time about it.

Thus, all types of studies have their advantages and disadvantages. The ultimate evaluation can be made only in view of many examples, preferably originating from many sources. Interim judgements must be made with caution. Practitioners should be prepared to be their own scientists, constantly monitoring their own choices of procedure, for both side effects and main effects.

LEGALITIES AND ETHICS

Some ethical issues have already been touched on in this chapter: the right of clients to withdraw from treatment, the obligation of practitioners to use the best treatment available, the necessity to report suspected abuse. A number of other ethical and legal issues are relevant to the social skills trainer. In many cases, the responsible person will be guided by the mandated ethical principles of his or her profession (e.g., American Psychological Association, 1981). The efforts of associations and lawyers to prevent ethical oversight have served well to establish basic working principles. However, the twilight zone remains, in which value judgements and conflicts of interest arise. The resolution of these cases can be difficult and painful.

Ultimately, all ethical principles are formulated in support of the question, "Is what is being done, or not being done, in the best interests of the child and of society?" The question is, obviously, not likely to produce a simple answer. Conflicts arise between the individual and society, and from our inability to determine "the best interests" with much degree of certainty. Again there is some pragmatic value in offering the child more choice. If the repertoire of responses is expanded, then a set of naturally balancing forces can remove the burden of godlike decisions from the shoulders of the childcare professional. That is, the child, with less limited options, will act in his or her own interests, and society will provide natural contingencies (reward or punishment, according to its interests) to the action.

An example of this solution is provided by the case of a boy with "cross gender" behaviors (Dowrick, 1983c), mentioned in Chapter 8 (p. 135). Rather than attempt value judgements of best interests based on the suppression of certain behavior, this 4-year-old boy was trained to *increase* his repertoire of public responses so that the social milieu naturally reinforced those actions that achieved his ends and were acceptable to society. (In short, he was taught to be as entertaining with junior engineer's kits and musical instruments as he already was with women's underwear and affective mannerisms.)

Below is a proposed set of ethical guidelines for the training of social skills with children. The principles are to some extent influenced by those developed for "assertive behavior training" (for adults) by Robert Alberti and others in 1976 (cited by Michelson et al., 1983, pp. 183–187) and by the ethical codes of the American Psychological Association (1981).

1) The fundamental purpose of training shall be to enlarge, not diminish, the repertoire of social initiations and responses available to the child.
2) Social skills trained shall be those that emphasize expressiveness (of thoughts and feelings) of the child, respectful of the rights of self, of others, and the cultural milieu.
3) Social skills are recognized as interpersonal and purposeful, and identified as behaviors that can be learned.
4) The child and caretaker shall give informed consent to the training. Being "informed" includes having:
   (a) descriptions of the types of anticipated experiences (e.g., role play, video recording);
   (b) descriptions of the potential effects and side effects;
   (c) reminders of rights to withdraw participation at any time;
   (d) evidence of qualifications of trainers, efficacy of the training package to be used, and suitability of the setting.
5) The child and caretaker shall be involved in self-determining aspects of training:
   (a) the child, to the extent possible, and the caretaker shall help develop and agree to objective goals of intervention;
   (b) the caretaker shall have access to materials and procedures.
6) The child's personal rights shall be protected in the following ways:

    (a) explicit and intelligible information on the conditions of confidentiality, agreed to by the child and caretaker;

    (b) additional steps to avoid coercion of children in an institutional environment.

7) Trainers of social skills will have appropriate qualifications:

    (a) with respect to the subject population. These qualifications are those generally applicable to the setting and age ranges of the children (e.g., preschool day care);

    (b) with respect to the general or incidental conditions (and disorders) of the trainees (e.g., delinquency, medical disorders);

    (c) with respect to training of social skills. These qualifications include a knowledge of the subject area, supervised experience in the development and application of training principles, and supervised training in the facilitation of groups.

8) The trainer shall be committed to offering training that is commensurate with the above qualifications, including a respect for the duration and comprehensiveness necessary for effective training, and a willingness to evaluate the immediate impact, generalization, and maintenance of effects.

9) The trainer shall have the ability and willingness to recognize the need to seek further resources and make referrals.

10) The trainer shall be guided by the ethical principles of his or her profession, and conduct all training within the law.

Communication Analysis –
Verbal and Nonverbal Skills

Observer: _____ Observee: _____ Date: _____

Rate the observed person *once* for each *component* listed, by circling the closest description available.

Check that you have made a total of 18 circles.

Add the number of circles in each column, and calculate scores as indicated.

Lower scores, obviously, are better.

(*Note*: Items 1–12 are *nonverbal*, 13–18 *verbal*. "Handing over" refers to cues and receptiveness to cues that enable the switching between talker and listener during conversation.)

Component	0	1	2
1. **face**	expressive	under expressive over expressive	blank v. exaggerated
2. **eye gaze**	mutual	little eye contact too much	quite averted staring
3. **posture**	relaxed	restless in place paces about	slumped rigid
4. **orientation**	centered	profile variable	turned away dominating

---

Developed by Peter W. Dowrick based on materials of Gabrielle M. Maxwell.

5. **responsiveness**	amiable	weak hyper	none excessive
6. **gestures**	expressive	very few too many/irrelevant	none wild
7. **voice volume**	firm	low variable	hardly audible very loud
8. **voice clarity**	clear	impeded variable	mumbled overly precise
9. **voice pitch**	varied	dull irrelevant	pure monotone exaggerated
10. **pace of speech**	varied	slow fast	interminable incomprehensible
11. **hesitation**	allows thought	variable without thought	stumbling overlap (relevant)
12. **handing over**	engaging	rambling interrupt (irrelevant)	says nothing dominates
13. **amount of speech**	moderate	too little too much	v. inadequate v. repetitive
14. **form of speech**	articulate	ungrammatical fluent errors	word salads very circular
15. **verbal sequences**	linked	pedantic hard to follow	v. predictable incomprehensible
16. **information content**	interesting	variable inaccurate	boring unbelievable
17. **emotional content**	stimulating	void uncomfortable	depressing hysterical
18. **verbal expressiveness**	suitable	variable flowery	none melodramatic

_____x 0=0   _____x 1=_____(B)   _____x 2=_____(C)

Total score (B+C)=_____

APPENDIX B

Standardized Assessments of Childhood Problems

Example

Walker Problem Behavior Identification Checklist
Revised 1976, by Hill M. Walker
Distributed by copyright holders, Western Psychological Services,
12031 Wilshire Blvd., Los Angeles, CA 90025

The checklist consists of 50 items, each of which contributes to one of five scales. It is usually responded to by a significant adult, on behalf of a child of elementary school age. The scales are:

1. Acting-out
2. Withdrawal
3. Distractibility
4. Disturbed Peer Relations
5. Immaturity

Instructions are to circle "the number to the right of the statement if you have observed that behavioral item in the child's response pattern during the last two month period." For copyright reasons, a sample only is printed here.

Sample items	Scale				
	1	2	3	4	5
1. Complains about others' unfairness and/or discrimination towards him.............3					
8. Other children act as if he were taboo or tainted..					4
11. Apologizes repeatedly for himself and/or his behavior.................................					2
14. Disturbs other children: teasing, provoking fights, interrupting others...........			2		
23. Utters nonsense syllables and/or babbles to himself...................................				4	
25. Comments that nobody likes him..........				2	
35. Openly strikes back with angry behavior to teasing of other children................3					
37. Has no friends..............................4					
42. Doesn't protest when others hurt, tease, or criticize him..............................3					
50. Frequently stares blankly into space and is unaware of his surroundings when doing so......1					

Circled items only are added to give column (scale) totals and an overall total. It will be seen that each item, when noted as present, contributes to one scale only, and that the weight of the contribution ranges 1–4. Thus, if a child is noted for items 8, 14, and 50, he or she would have a score of 4 on Scale 5, but only 3 on Scale 3.

Obtained scores may be compared with normalized scores of other children. Boys typically score much higher on Acting-out, Distractibility, and Disturbed Peer Relations scales, somewhat higher on Immaturity, and much the same as girls on Withdrawal. Comparison with norms allows verification of problem areas and suitability of social survival training. The individual scores can also be used as part of before and after measures, to assess the impact of treatment.

APPENDIX C

Ryall and Dietiker Fear Survey

CHILDREN'S FEAR SURVEY SCHEDULE ITEMS

Each item is answered on a 3 point scale as follows: 0=not (afraid)(scared)(nervous);
1=a little (afraid)(scared)(nervous); 2=very (afraid)(scared)(nervous)

1. Loud noises	0..1..2	26. Storms	0..1..2
2. Bugs	0..1..2	27. Graveyards	0..1..2
3. Fire	0..1..2	28. The principal	0..1..2
4. Teachers	0..1..2	29. Lions and tigers	0..1..2
5. Snakes	0..1..2	30. Dark, empty rooms	0..1..2
6. Being alone	0..1..2	31. Guns	0..1..2
7. Spankings	0..1..2	32. Dad	0..1..2
8. Strangers	0..1..2	33. Being sick	0..1..2
9. Dogs	0..1..2	34. Mom shouting	0..1..2
10. To die	0..1..2	35. Going to the dentist	0..1..2
11. Earthquakes	0..1..2	36. Monsters	0..1..2
12. Brothers	0..1..2	37. Cats	0..1..2
13. Spiders	0..1..2	38. Shadows	0..1..2
14. To get hurt	0..1..2	39. Sharks	0..1..2
15. Haunted houses	0..1..2	40. Ghosts	0..1..2
16. Grades on report cards	0..1..2	41. Being bawled out	0..1..2
17. Death or dead people	0..1..2	42. Poison	0..1..2
18. Closed in places	0..1..2	43. Seeing other kids fight	0..1..2
19. Getting caught	0..1..2	44. Going to the doctor	0..1..2
20. Being in a fight	0..1..2	45. Scary movies	0..1..2
21. Kidnappers	0..1..2	46. Bears	0..1..2
22. Grades on tests	0..1..2	47. War	0..1..2
23. The dark	0..1..2	48. Bad dreams	0..1..2
24. Big bullies	0..1..2	49. Anything else	0..1..2
25. Getting a shot	0..1..2	50. Anything else	0..1..2

From Ryall & Dietiker, 1979, reprinted with permission. Copyright 1979, Pergamon Press Ltd.

APPENDIX D

Assessment of Parent-Child Interactions

An assessment system based on the Budd System (Budd & Fabry, 1984; Budd, Riner, & Brockman, 1983) provides a method for obtaining essential data to implement intervention planning, allowing meaningful outcome measurements, without unreasonable cost in terms of time. The system consists of five brief, structured activities, aimed at different, potential training strategies. The parent skills assessed are evidently the most important in providing the clarity and consistency of communication necessary for children to feel secure and guided within the family system. They embody many of the skills identified for adults seeking rapport with children. Ideally, assessments occur in the family's home, but may be made elsewhere, as long as both parent and child can be present. Observers will need a stop watch, and a clipboard with observation sheets prepared for quick scoring on the basis of the five separate categories of skill. A watch, calculator, or other instrument that can be set to make an unobtrusive tone once per minute is also useful. Each of the five assessment tasks takes between 10 and 20 minutes.

Instruct parents on each task. Ask them to repeat their understanding of the instructions for verification. If an assessment task goes awry, simply start again, following clarification.

I. INSTRUCTION GIVING – Parents are observed and scored during the performance of five separate observable tasks which they have devised. These tasks are to be ones of which the child is known to be capable, but not chores which the child dislikes.

II. DIFFERENTIAL ATTENTION—Parents are observed and scored for 5-minute period, during which time the parent is asked to do some solitary activity while the child is asked to play independently. The parent is instructed that every minute there will be an audible tone, at which she or he may choose whether or not to interact with the child. However, the rest of the time interactions are to be kept at a minimum.

III. USE OF CONTINGENCIES—Parents are observed and scored for a 5-minute period, during which time the parent is asked to direct the child in a chore, using a point system for structured payoffs.

IV. TEACHING NEW SKILLS—Parents are observed and scored for five separate periods of 1 to 2 minutes each. During these short time periods, the parents are asked to direct the child in the practice of new tasks. (Although the observations are very similar to those in IN-STRUCTION GIVING, the demands on parent and child are different, involving new rather than familiar tasks.)

VI. USE OF TIME OUT—Parents are observed and scored while being asked to roleplay the use of time out. Explanations are given to both the parent and child stating that the task involves "play-acting" what happens when the child does something naughty.

The observation scoring sheets on the following pages are for families of children 8 to 12 years old. They reflect the published observational strategies of Budd and Fabry (1984), devised for younger children. The scoring method was devised by Peter W. Dowrick, assisted by Donna Teekell and Linda Lenoir.

INSTRUCTION GIVING

Parents devise five observable tasks, estimated to take about 2 to 3 minutes each. These tasks should be ones of which the child is known to be capable, but not that the child dislikes; for example: feeding the cat; looking to see if the mail has arrived. For each task, the following observations are made.

Observations: *Task#*

	1	2	3	4	5
1) Brief description of task					
2) Estimated time for task					
3) Record Y or N (yes or no) for each of the following:					
a) Parent gets child's attention	Y N	Y N	Y N	Y N	Y N
b) Parent gives clear instruction .... (a directive – free of reproach)	Y N	Y N	Y N	Y N	Y N
c) Child begins within 10 secs	Y N	Y N	Y N	Y N	Y N
d) Parent waits (quiet) 10 secs or more	Y N	Y N	Y N	Y N	Y N
If child not begin within first 10 secs: e) Parent repeats instruction............	Y N	Y N	Y N	Y N	Y N
f) Child begins within next 10 secs	Y N	Y N	Y N	Y N	Y N
g) Parent helps within 30 secs of last instruction	Y N	Y N	Y N	Y N	Y N
h) Parent helps after 30 secs of last instruction	Y N	Y N	Y N	Y N	Y N
i) Child begins with help	Y N	Y N	Y N	Y N	Y N
j) Child finishes independently	Y N	Y N	Y N	Y N	Y N
k) Child finishes with help	Y N	Y N	Y N	Y N	Y N
l) Parent positively comments on child's behavior	Y N	Y N	Y N	Y N	Y N
m) Parent negatively comments on child's behavior	Y N	Y N	Y N	Y N	Y N
n) Child communicates resistance to task	Y N	Y N	Y N	Y N	Y N
o) Child communicates positively to parent	Y N	Y N	Y N	Y N	Y N
4) Record duration of trial.........................					

Notes:

DIFFERENTIAL ATTENTION

The parent is requested to do some solitary activity for 5 minutes or more (such as reading, letter writing, paperwork), and to ask his or her child to play independently in the meantime. The parent is told that every minute there will be an audible tone and "You may or may not choose to interact with (child's name) at the tone. The rest of the time, please keep your interactions to a minimum."

Observation:

At each tone, make three recordings, based on activity during the past 60 seconds.

Tone#

	1	2	3	4	5	6	7	8	9	10
1) Check *one* – parent behavior (most recent):										
a) praises										
b) ignores										
c) requests										
d) describes										
e) disapproves										
f) other										
g) none										
2) Check *one* – child behavior: a) independent										
b) interactive....................................										
3) Record Y *or* N (yes or no) for child interferences:										

Notes:

USE OF CONTINGENCIES

The parent is asked to direct the child in a 5-minute chore (e.g., tidy part of bedroom) using a point system for structured payoffs. Many parents may already be familiar with using a point system without training. But if not, the task can be described thus: "You can offer your child a reward for doing (chore). You should let (child's name) earn the reward by getting a total number of points – you can give points to him/her for doing specific parts of the job." For younger children, stars, etc., may be more appropriate. Answer any questions the parent may have.

Observations:

Record observations in three phases. Phase two will be recorded 6 times (once every 60 secs at the tone) unless the task is completed sooner. If task takes over 6 minutes, wait to record phase three.

1) Preparation:
   a) Parent sets up point display .... Y N
   b) Explains point system to child .... Y N
   c) Negotiates reward with child .... Y N
   d) Negotiates criterion with child .... Y N
2) At every 60 secs at the tone,
   record Y or N (yes or no):

Tone#

	1	2	3	4	5	6
a) Parent gave points in last 60 secs	Y N	Y N	Y N	Y N	Y N	Y N
b) Points given appropriate to arranged contingency	Y N	Y N	Y N	Y N	Y N	Y N
c) Points given accompanied with praise	Y N	Y N	Y N	Y N	Y N	Y N
d) Parent took points off in last 60 secs	Y N	Y N	Y N	Y N	Y N	Y N

e) Points deducted appropriate to arranged contingency	Y N	Y N	Y N	Y N	Y N	Y N
f) Points deducted accompanied with explanation	Y N	Y N	Y N	Y N	Y N	Y N
g) Child on task (at tone)	Y N	Y N	Y N	Y N	Y N	Y N

3) Completion – Record Y or N (yes or no) at completion:
   a) Parent asks child or helps child to tally points .... Y N
   b) Parent explains whether or not the points earn reward ..... Y N
   c) Parent gives descriptive appraisal for future .... Y N
   d) Parent rewards according to criterion .... Y N

Notes:

TEACHING NEW SKILLS

The parent is asked to direct the child in the practice of new tasks (e.g., a new crochet stitch; a new chord on the guitar). Five simple tasks, 1 to 2 minutes each, are called for.

Observations:

	Task #				
	1	2	3	4	5
1) Brief description of task					
2) Record P (done by parent) *or* C (done by child) *or* −D (not done) *or* −N (not applicable)					
a) Distractions removed (e.g. TV off)	P C −D −N	P C −D −N	P C −D −N	P C −D −N	P C −D −N
b) Appropriate materials selected	P C −D −N	P C −D −N	P C −D −N	P C −D −N	P C −D −N
3) Record Y or N (yes or no) c) Parent gets child's attention ...	Y N	Y N	Y N	Y N	Y N
d) Parent gives clear instruction	Y N	Y N	Y N	Y N	Y N
e) Parent models the skill	Y N	Y N	Y N	Y N	Y N

f) Child begins within 10 secs	Y N	Y N	Y N	Y N	Y N
g) Parent waits quietly for 10 secs or more	Y N	Y N	Y N	Y N	Y N
If child not begin in first 10 seconds: h) Parent repeats instruction ...	Y N	Y N	Y N	Y N	Y N
i) Child begins within next 10 seconds	Y N	Y N	Y N	Y N	Y N
j) Parent helps within 30 secs of last instruction	Y N	Y N	Y N	Y N	Y N
k) Parent helps after 30 seconds of last instruction	Y N	Y N	Y N	Y N	Y N
l) Child begins with help	Y N	Y N	Y N	Y N	Y N
m) Parent praises descriptively	Y N	Y N	Y N	Y N	Y N
n) Child finishes independently ...	Y N	Y N	Y N	Y N	Y N
o) Child finishes with help	Y N	Y N	Y N	Y N	Y N
p) Parent negatively comments on child's behavior	Y N	Y N	Y N	Y N	Y N
q) Child communicates resistance to task	Y N	Y N	Y N	Y N	Y N
r) Child communicates positively to parent	Y N	Y N	Y N	Y N	Y N

Notes:

USE OF TIME OUT

Parent and child are asked to role-play the use of timeout. If the parent needs an explanation, say: "This is like sending the kid to the bedroom, or some undesirable spot, for a period of time for being naughty." If the parent has some experience with time out, s/he is asked to act as if these were new circumstances. It is explained to the child that we are going to play act what happens when s/he does something wrong.

Observations:

Record Y or N (yes or no) for each item in the four phases:

1) Explanation
   a) Parent explains what is to be timed out .... Y N
   b) Child agrees .... Y N
   c) Parent names the time out area .... Y N
   d) Parent explains what is to be done in time out .... Y N
   e) Parent explains exit criteria .... Y N
2) Misbehavior
   a) Parent names the misbehavior .... Y N
   b) Parent avoids recriminations .... Y N
   c) Chosen time out area is less engaging than present situa-
      tion .... Y N
   d) Parent guides child to time out .... Y N
   e) Parent states time for time out, sets timer .... Y N
3) Time out
   a) Child leaves time out inappropriately .... Y N
   b) If (a), parent restates rule .... Y N
   c) If (a), parent resets timer .... Y N
   d) Child acts out in time out area .... Y N
   e) If (d), parent resets timer .... Y N
   f) Parent makes no other comments or recriminations .... Y N
4) Closure
   a) Parent announces end of time out .... Y N
   b) Time out lasted time agreed .... Y N
   c) Parent makes no recriminations .... Y N
   d) Parent offers positive attention (within 2 mins) .... Y N

Notes:

A P P E N D I X E

Social Survival

Situation Analysis

Form 1   Date _____
Filled in for _____ by _____ Before/After

Degree of difficulty

Here are some situations that people often find difficult to deal with. Please read each item, and mark the column that you think would apply to you *at the present time*.	*Not at all difficult*	*A little bit difficult*	*Sometimes easy sometimes hard*	*Very difficult*	*Extremely difficult*
1. Do you find it difficult to introduce someone to someone else?					
2. Do you find it difficult making conversation with friends or people you know?					
3. Do you find it difficult making conversation with strangers?					
4. Do you find it difficult talking to someone of the opposite sex?					
5. Do you find it difficult having to say something in a group of people?					
6. Do you find it difficult to call a business (e.g., bus timetable inquiry) on the telephone?					

Adapted by Peter W. Dowrick and Marie Hood for developmentally disabled teenagers and young adults from assertiveness training materials of John M. Raeburn.

7. Do you find it difficult buying things in a store?					
8. Do you find it difficult making a complaint, e.g., about the behavior of a classmate/workmate, or about something you have bought?					
9. Do you find it difficult sorting out your problems at a Social Services Department or similar place?					
10. Do you find it difficult getting along with any of your classmates/workmates?					
11. Do you find it difficult getting along with any one person in your family?					
12. Do you find it difficult to ask for a favor or anything else from a teacher/supervisor?					
13. Do you find it difficult to ask for information or help from "important" people such as Principal, Doctor, Bus-Driver, or Foreman?					
14. Do you find it difficult to disagree with anybody, even if you are right?					
15. Do you find it difficult telling someone off?					
16. Do you find it difficult to stand up for yourself when someone is being pushy?					
17. Do you find it difficult if a teacher/supervisor criticizes your work?					
18. Do you find it difficult if someone of your age criticizes you?					
19. Do you find it difficult showing anger to someone you are angry with?					
20. Do you find it difficult having an interview (e.g., job interview)?					
21. What are two other situations you find very or extremely difficult? 1. _____ . 2. _____ .					

Bibliography: Annotations of Selected Materials

Materials selected for description include nearly 40 books, two special issues of journals, and two videotape training packages published between 1979 and 1985. A small number of items are specifically devoted to social skills and children. Other materials present research and procedures for the retraining of children's social deficits (but described in other terms). Several books contain pertinent chapters in the context of a larger topic, or deal with issues apparently relevant to, but so far absent from, the social skills and children literature.

The bibliography is by no means exhaustive. However, because serious attention to the field has been applied so recently, the list, I hope, should be highly representative. In some cases, comparable works exist as worthy alternatives to those noted. My commentaries are intended to be informative, not evaluative. They are based partly on an earlier publication (Dowrick, P. W., & Gilligan, C. A. Social skills and children: An annotated bibliography. *The Behavior Therapist*, 1985, *8*, 211-213).

239

Argyle, M., & Trower, P. (1979). *Person to person: Ways of communication.* New York: Harper & Row.

Highly illustrated, detailed discussion of verbal and nonverbal communication in adults. A comparable book for children would be valuable.

Asher, S. R., & Gottman, J. M. (Eds.). (1981). *The development of children's friendships.* Cambridge: Cambridge University Press.

Twelve chapters, emphasizing research. Part I, "Group processes," includes assessment, social structure of popularity and friendship, and differences within or between groups (interracial; mental retardation). Part II, "Social-cognitive processes," contains one chapter on training social skills, others analyzing naturally occurring processes.

Bellack, A. S., & Hersen, M. (Eds.). (1979). *Research and practice in social skills training.* New York: Plenum Press.

The social psychology of social skills techniques and development, verbal and nonverbal communication, and theoretical models. One chapter only on children, which reviews the research on social skills training and assessment. A related chapter includes the development of psychopathology.

Buss, A. H. (1980). *Self-consciousness and social anxiety.* San Francisco: W. H. Freeman.

A theory of self-consciousness and its implications. Basic components and examples are provided for social skills training with children, adolescents, and handicapped children. Discussions include the selection of social skills, assessment, teaching process, generalization, and maintenance. One chapter specifically addresses "shyness."

Camp, B.W., & Bash, M.A.S. (1985). *Think aloud: Increasing social and cognitive skills—A problem solving program for children.* Champaign, IL: Research Press.

Three manuals for classroom use: grades 1–2; 3–4; 5–6. Each manual contains procedures for training social survival strategies, following the problem solving approach previously developed by the authors. Each manual may be purchased independently, and contains age-appropriate scripts and forms.

Cartledge, G., & Milburn, J. (Eds.). (1985). *Teaching social skills to children: Innovative approaches* (2nd ed.). New York: Pergamon Press.

Social skills training oriented to a school curriculum. Part I, by the editors, sets out general assessment and teaching procedures. In Part II, contributions by different authors, one chapter describes cooperation training, others focus on specific populations: behavior disorders (aggression, withdrawal); handicap; young children; adolescents.

Curran, J. P., & Monti, P. M. (Eds.). (1982). *Social skills treatment: A practical handbook for assessment and treatment.* New York: Guilford Press.

One chapter on children with peer relationship difficulties. The book addresses a variety of other populations, with particular emphasis on schizophrenia and influencing variables, such as family.

Dangel, R. F., & Polster, R. A. (Eds.). (1984). *Parent training: Foundations of research and practice.* New York: Guilford Press.

Twenty comprehensive chapters on parenting, with a behavioral emphasis.

A research-based treatise in helping parents to communicate with children of different populations.

Eisler, R. M., & Fredriksen, L. W. (1980). *Perfecting social skills: A guide to interpersonal behavior development.* New York: Plenum Press.
    A theoretical framework for the development of social skills, their effects, and the basic principles of training. Research examples emphasize practical application; Chapter 8: "Skills training with children."

Goldstein, A. P., Sprafkin, R. P., Gershaw, N. J., & Klein, P. (1980). *Skillstreaming the adolescent: A structured-learning approach to teaching prosocial skills.* Champaign, IL: Research Press.
    A training program package. Initial chapters outline the procedures and their rationale; checklist assessments are provided. Later chapters give details of target skills, with trainer notes and example dialogues with trainees. A book using similar procedures for younger children is also available (McGinnis, E., & Goldstein, A. P. (1984). *Skillstreaming the elementary school child: A guide to teaching prosocial skills).*

Graziano, A. M., & Mooney, K. C. (1984). *Children and behavior therapy.* New York: Aldine.
    A review of the major developments in child behavior therapy during 1975–1981. Social skills training is not addressed although related issues are: autistic children, mentally retarded children, children's control of fear, behavioral self-control, juvenile delinquency, family systems, and intervention in school.

Hamerlynck, L. A. (Ed.). (1979). *Behavioral systems for the developmentally disabled: (Vol. 1). School and family environments.* New York: Brunner/Mazel.
    One chapter specifically on social survival. Chapter 4, "PEERS: A program for remediating social withdrawal in school," describes the development and procedures of a standardized intervention program for young elementary school children in the regular classroom.

Hargie, O., Saunders, C., & Dickson, D. (1981). *Social skills in interpersonal communication.* London: Croom Helm.
    Communication principles for professional interaction with adult clients (could be usefully adapted for children). Chapter-length descriptions of training procedures in: nonverbal communication, reinforcement, questioning, reflecting, set-induction and closure, explaining, listening, and self-disclosure.

Hazel, J. S., Schumaker, J. B., Sherman, J. A., & Sheldon-Wildgen, J. (1983). *ASSET: Adolescent social skills evaluation and training.* Champaign, IL: Research Press.
    Videotape integrated package for group training. A series of modules in eight skill areas (e.g., giving and receiving negative feedback, resisting peer pressure) with stimulus and modeling videotapes (or films) designed for young adolescents.

Jackson, N. F., Jackson, D. A., & Monroe, S. (1983). *Getting along with others: Teaching social effectiveness to children.* Champaign, IL: Research Press.
    Applicable to regular elementary school classrooms. In two volumes (available separately or as a set), one details scripts and activities for group sessions to train a variety of social skills (e.g., self-introduction, saying no, compromising). The other volume is a program guide containing rationale and global training strategies.

Jones, W. H., Cheek, J. M., & Briggs, S. R. (Eds.). (1985). *Shyness: Perspectives on research and treatment*. New York: Plenum Press.
A sizeable volume emphasizing the phenomenology of shyness. Includes three chapters on the development of shyness in children, and five short chapters on interventions, largely relevant to adults.

Journal of Pediatric Psychology. (1981). (Special section on children's social skills), *6*, 335–434.
Six articles covering normative and developmental issues, learning disabilities, and peer intervention strategies.

Karoly, P., & Steffen, J. J. (Eds.). (1982). *Improving children's competence: Advances in child behavioral analysis and therapy*. Lexington, MA: D. C. Heath.
One chapter on concepts of social competence; others describing procedures and research evaluation. One chapter concerns social skills training for socially withdrawn children, others provide a variety of approaches to different skills for developmentally disabled children. Also by the same editors is a book concerning older children (*Adolescent behavior disorders: Foundations and contemporary concerns*, 1984). It has two chapters that describe assessment of social competence, and communication training in families.

Kelly, J. A. (1982). *Social skills training: A practical guide for interventions*. New York: Springer.
Divided equally between chapters on general principles and procedures, and chapters on specific skills. One chapter on social skills for children (describes components, procedures, and some studies).

Kent, M. W., & Rolf, J. E. (Eds.). (1979). *Primary prevention of psychopathology, Vol. 3: Social competence in children*. Hanover, NH: University Press of New England.
Proceedings of a conference. Two chapters describe programs for training children's interpersonal problem solving ability (one for mothers, the other for teachers). Most of the other 11 chapters discuss factors that influence the development of competence, or the implications of a lack of competence.

Kratochwill, T. R. (1981). *Selective mutism: Implications for research and treatment*. Hillsdale, NJ: Lawrence Erlbaum.
Review of theory and research on selective mutism. Four chapters provide overviews of different approaches to this communication disorder. Three chapters describe current behavioral interventions in detail, and ideas on the future of treatment are presented.

L'Abate, L., & Milan, M. A. (Eds.). (1985). *Handbook of social skills training and research*. Chichester: Wiley.
A large volume on the origins and applications of social skills training for a wide variety of populations. Content emphasis is upon adults, but chapters include reference to children, parents, and developmentally disabled.

Lahey, B. B., & Kazdin, A. E. (Eds.). (1981). *Advances in clinical child psychology* (Vol. 4). New York: Plenum Press.
Two chapters with specific relevance to social survival. "Social skills assessment of children" reviews theoretical, conceptual, methodological, psychometric, and programmatic issues. "Peers as behavior change agents for withdrawn

classmates" reviews procedures and research findings on systematic and incidental influence by children on their shy peers. Other chapters have some relevance to social function. A later book in the same series (Vol. 6, 1983) includes a chapter that reviews training for children with peer problems: "Social relationship problems in children: An approach to intervention."

Mash, E. J., & Terdal, L. G. (Eds.). (1981). *Behavioral assessment of childhood disorders*. New York: Guilford Press.

Chapter 8 – "Social skills deficits." Several other chapters are relevant to assessment in social problems of children (e.g., conduct problems; fears; gender problems; obesity).

Michelson, L., Sugai, D. P., Wood, R. P., & Kazdin, A. (1983). *Social skills assessment and training with children: An empirically based handbook*. New York: Plenum Press.

Assessment and program implementation details for social skills training with aggressive or withdrawn children. Relevant findings on social development and empirical studies of intervention are briefly reviewed, followed by details of 16 training modules and associated materials.

Morris, R. J., & Kratochwill, T. J. (Eds.). (1983). *The practice of child therapy*. New York: Pergamon Press.

Eleven contributed chapters on a variety of childhood disorders and their treatment (behavioral emphasis). The four chapters most relevant to social skills: fears; communication disorders; aggression; delinquency.

Patterson, G. R. (1982). *Coercive family process*. Eugene, OR: Castalia Publishing.

Extensive and detailed review of childhood aggression. Substantial theory and research, focusing on reciprocal effects within the family, are presented. One chapter describes family treatment (emphasis on behavioral parent training), and one relates aggression to other antisocial behavior.

Patterson, M. L. (1983). *Nonverbal behavior: A functional perspective*. New York: Springer-Verlag.

Examination of the social function of adult nonverbal behavior. The book reviews the goals or purposes served by patterns of nonverbal behaviors, discusses the role of nonverbal behavior in social exchange.

Ross, A. O. (1981). *Child behavior therapy: Principles, procedures, and empirical bases*. New York: Wiley.

Review and summary of principles on which behavioral treatment of children is based. Chapters are arranged by type of disorder, classified as behavioral deficits or behavioral excesses. A social skills training approach is taken to social withdrawal.

Rubin, K. H., & Ross, H. S. (Eds.). (1982). *Peer relationships and social skills in childhood*. New York: Springer-Verlag.

A detailed examination of social skills and peer relationships across the full spectrum of age groups and selected special populations. Part I describes developmental aspects of prosocial behavior. Part II focuses predominantly on peer relationships. Part III examines individual differences in peer relationships and social skills.

Schaeffer, C. E., Johnson, L., & Wherry, J. N. (1982). *Group therapies for children and youth*. San Francisco: Jossey-Bass.
A collection of short procedural descriptions (mostly case studies). Condensed articles on shyness, fears, aggression, poor peer relations, delinquency, and other problems illustrate a wide variety of approaches. Other books by Schaefer and colleagues, containing case studies in digest form, are available from the same publisher.

Schinke, S. P., & Gilchrist, L. D. (1984). *Life skills with adolescents*. Baltimore: University Park Press.
A behavioral counseling approach to the life skills a child should acquire before adult autonomy. Areas addressed include: interpersonal relationships, sexuality, stress and health, work and society.

Schloss, P. J. (1983). *Social development of handicapped children and adolescents*. Rockville, MD: Aspen Systems.
Framework for and description of intervention strategies. Provides a social learning approach, and offers some considerations for handicapped populations.

Social skills training for children. (1983). *Child and Youth Services* (Special issue), *5* (3,4).
Eight articles on a variety of topics. Issues raised: early development; applicability of research. Two general approaches are described: cognitive-social-learning; classroom settings. Populations specifically dealt with: withdrawn children; adolescents; court adjudicated youth; emotionally disturbed adolescents.

Spence, S., & Shepherd, G. (Eds.). (1983). *Developments in social skills training*. New York: Academic Press.
A variety of issues and interventions (mostly institution based). Section II, "Social skills training with children and adolescents," includes three chapters, which focus on school children, adolescent psychiatric outpatients, and adolescent offenders.

Stephens, T. M., Hartman, A. C., & Lucas, V. H. (1982). *Teaching children basic skills: A curriculum handbook*. Columbus, OH: Charles E. Merrill.
A guide to teaching mildly handicapped children, elementary school age, academic (six parts) and social (one part) skills. Detailed curriculum objectives are provided, with sample assessment and teaching strategies. The guide reflects an earlier work by Stephens: *Social skills in the classroom*. Columbus, OH: Cedar Press, 1978.

Strain, P. S. (Ed.). (1981). *The utilization of classroom peers as behavior change agents*. New York: Plenum Press.
A review of peer relationships, and their incidental and programmatic influence on children's educational and social development. Two chapters have procedures for withdrawal and aggression; others address methodology and specific populations. A book of related interest written by Strain is: *Social development of exceptional children*, Rockville, MD: Aspen Systems.

Varni, J. W. (1983). *Clinical behavioral pediatrics*. New York: Pergamon Press.
One chapter on childhood social skills deficits, recognizing the synergy be-

tween social behavior and health. A recent trend in books on different childhood disorders is to include some reference to factors of interpersonal functioning.

Walker, H. M., McConnell, S., Holmes, D., Todis, B., Walker, J., & Golden, J. (1983). *The Walker social skills curriculum: The ACCEPTS program.* Austin, TX, Pro-Ed.

A packaged social skills program aimed at and developed for the handicapped child mainstreamed in the public school (primary and intermediate grades). Step-by-step instructions for individual training, assessments, reinforcement strategies, and modeling situations are provided. The manual may be used on its own, or in conjunction with videotaped stimulus and modeling materials.

Wine, J. D., & Smye, M. D. (Eds.). (1981). *Social competence.* New York: Guilford Press.

Two chapters on children's issues: sociometric and behavioral assessment; social problem solving. Other chapters provide contrasting conceptualizations and procedures for specific adult populations.

Zimbardo, P. G. (1985). *Shyness: What it is, what to do about it* (2nd ed.). Menlo Park, CA: Addison-Wesley.

Simple tactics and strategies for social effectiveness, primarily as self-help for adults, but also oriented to children. Examines different types of shyness, problems faced by shy individuals, and the origins and analysis of shyness. Explores shyness as implicated in alcoholism, criminality, and sexual disorders. How-to chapters include "Building your self-esteem," "Developing your social skills."

References

Alberti, R. E., & Emmons, M. L. (1974). *Your perfect right: A guide to asser-tive behavior* (2nd ed.). San Luis Obispo, CA: Impact Press.

Alexander, J. F. (1974). Behavior modification and delinquent youth. In J. C. Cull & R. E. Hardy (Eds.), *Behavior modification in rehabilitation settings.* Springfield, IL: Charles C Thomas.

Alexander, J. F., Barton, C., Schiavo, R. S., & Parsons, B. V. (1976). Systems-behavioral intervention with families of delinquents: Therapist characteristics, family behavior, and outcome. *Journal of Consulting and Clinical Psychology, 44,* 656–664.

American Psychological Association (1981). Ethical principles of psychologists (rev. ed.). *American Psychologist, 36,* 633–638.

Argyle, M. (1964). *Psychology and social problems.* London: Methuen.

Arkowitz, H., Lichenstein, E., McGovern, K., & Hines, P. (1975). The behavioral assessment of social competence in males. *Behavior Therapy, 6,* 3–13.

Arsenio, W. F. (1983, August). *The role of affect in children's understanding of social rules.* Paper presented at 91st Annual Convention of American Psychological Association, Anaheim.

Asher, S. R., & Hymel, S. (1981). Children's social competence in peer relations: Sociometric and behavioral assessment. In J. D. Wine & M. D. Smye (Eds.), *Social competence* (pp. 125–157). New York: Guilford Press.

Asher, S. R., Singleton, L. C., Tinsley, B. R., & Hymel, S. (1979). A reliable sociometric measure for preschool children. *Developmental Psychology, 15,* 443–444.

Axelrod, S., & Apsche, J. (Eds.). (1983). *The effects of punishment on human behavior.* New York: Academic Press.

Azrin, N. H., Sneed, T. J., & Foxx, R. M. (1974). Drybed training: Rapid elimina-tion of childhood enuresis. *Behaviour Research and Therapy, 12,* 147–156.

247

Baer, D. M. (1981). *How to plan for generalization.* Lawrence, KS: H & H Enterprises.

Baer, R. A., Williams, J. A., Osnes, P. G., & Stokes, T. F. (1984). Delayed reinforcement as an indiscriminable contingency in verbal/nonverbal correspondence training. *Journal of Applied Behavior Analysis, 17,* 429–440.

Bandura, A. (1969). *Principles of behavior modification.* New York: Holt, Rinehart & Winston.

Bandura, A. (1973). *Aggression: A social learning analysis.* Englewood Cliffs, NJ: Prentice-Hall.

Bandura, A. (1977a). Self-efficacy: Towards a unifying theory of behavioral change. *Psychological Review, 84,* 191–215.

Bandura, A. (1977b). *Social learning theory.* Englewood Cliffs, NJ: Prentice-Hall.

Bandura, A. (1986). *Social foundations of thought and action: A social cognitive theory.* Englewood Cliffs, NJ: Prentice-Hall.

Bandura, A., Ross, D., & Ross, S. A. (1963). Imitation in film-mediated aggressive models. *Journal of Abnormal and Social Psychology, 66,* 3–11.

Barkley, R. (1981). *Hyperactive children: A handbook for diagnosis and treatment.* New York: Guilford Press.

Barkley, R. (1983). Hyperactivity. In R. J. Morris & T. R. Kratochwill (Eds.), *The practice of child therapy* (pp. 87–112). New York: Pergamon Press.

Barrios, B. A., Hartmann, D. P., & Shigetomi, C. (1981). Fears and anxieties in children. In E. J. Mash & L. G. Terdal (Eds.), *Behavioral assessment of childhood disorders* (pp. 259–304). New York: Guilford Press.

Bash, M. A. S., & Camp, B. W. (1980). Teacher training in the think aloud classroom program. In G. Cartledge & J. F. Milburn (Eds.), *Teaching social skills to children: Innovative approaches* (pp. 143–178). New York: Pergamon Press.

Bateson, G., Jackson, D. D., Haley, J., & Weakland, J. H. (1956). Toward a theory of schizophrenia. *Behavioral Science, 1,* 251–264.

Beck, A. T. (1976). *Cognitive therapy and the emotional disorders.* New York: International Universities Press.

Becker, W. C. (1971). *Parents are teachers: A child management program.* Champaign, IL: Research Press.

Bernal, M. E. (1984). Consumer issues in parent training. In R. F. Dangel & R. A. Polster (Eds.), *Parent-training: Foundations of research and practice* (pp. 477–503). New York: Guilford Press.

Betts, T. (1983). Developing a videotape library. In P. W. Dowrick & S. J. Biggs (Eds.), *Using video: Psychological and social applications* (pp. 61–71). Chichester: Wiley.

Bornstein, M. R., Bellack, A. S., & Hersen, M. (1977). Social skills training for unassertive children: A multiple baseline analysis. *Journal of Applied Behavior Analysis, 10,* 183–195.

Brady, J. P. (1984). Social skills training for psychiatric patients, II: Clinical outcome studies. *American Journal of Psychiatry, 141,* 491–498.

Budd, K. S., & Fabry, P. L. (1984). Behavioral assessment in applied parent training: Use of a structured observation system. In R. F. Dangel & R. A. Polster (Eds.), *Parent training: Foundations of research and practice* (pp. 417–442). New York: Guilford Press.

Budd, K. S., Riner, L. S., & Brockman, M. P. (1983). A structured observation system for clinical evaluation of parent training. *Behavioral Assessment, 5,* 373–393.

Burchard, J. D., & Lane, T. W. (1982). Crime and delinquency. In A. S. Bellack, M. Hersen, & A. E. Kazdin (Eds.), *International handbook of behavior modification and therapy* (pp. 613–652). New York: Plenum Press.

Burnett, J. M. (1978). Training emotionally disturbed children in assertive behavior (Doctoral dissertation, Southern Illinois University at Carbondale, 1978). *Dissertation Abstracts International, 39,* 1944B.

Camp, B. W. (1977). Verbal mediation in young aggressive boys. *Journal of Abnormal Psychology, 86,* 145–153.

Camp, B. W., Blom, G. E., Herbert, F., & Van Doorninck, W. J. (1977). "Think Aloud": A program for developing self-control in young aggressive boys. *Journal of Abnormal Child Psychology, 5,* 157–169.

Campbell, D. T., & Stanley, J. C. (1966). *Experimental and quasi-experimental designs for research.* Chicago: Rand McNally.

Campbell, S. B., & Cluss, P. (1982). Peer relationships of young children with behavior problems. In K. H. Rubin & H. S. Ross (Eds.), *Peer relationships and social skills in childhood.* New York: Springer-Verlag.

Caplan, G. (1961). *Prevention of mental disorders in children: Initial explorations.* New York: Basic Books.

Carden-Smith, L. K., & Fowler, S. A. (1984). Positive peer pressure: The effects of peer monitoring on children's disruptive behavior. *Journal of Applied Behavior Analysis, 17,* 213–227.

Carr, E. G. (1980). Generalization of treatment effects following educational intervention with autistic children and youth. In B. Wilcox & A. Thompson (Eds.), *Critical issues in educating autistic children and youth.* Washington, DC: U. S. Department of Education, Office of Special Education.

Carr, E. G. (1985). Behavioral approaches to language and communication. In E. Schopter & G. Mesibov (Eds.), *Current issues in autism: Vol. III. Communication problems in autism* (pp. 37–57). New York: Plenum Press.

Carr, E. G., & Durand, V. M. (1985). Reducing behavior problems through functional communication training. *Journal of Applied Behavior Analysis, 18,* 111–126.

Carrol, W. R., & Bandura, A. (1982). The role of visual monitoring in observational learning of action patterns: Making the unobservable observable. *Journal of Motor Behavior, 14,* 153–167.

Cartledge, G., & Milburn, J. F. (1978). The case for teaching social skills in the classroom: A review. *Review of Educational Research, 1,* 133–156.

Cartledge, G., & Milburn, J. F. (1980). *Teaching social skills to children: Innovative approaches.* New York: Pergamon Press.

Castenada, A., McCandless, B., & Palermo, D. (1956). The children's form of the Manifest Anxiety Scale. *Child Development, 27,* 317–326.

Cautela, J. R., & Baron, M. G. (1977). Covert conditioning: A theoretical analysis. *Behavior Modification, 1,* 351–368.

Chapman, C., & Risley, T. R. (1974). Anti-litter procedures in an urban high-density area. *Journal of Applied Behavior Analysis, 7,* 377–383.

Christophersen, E. R. (1984). *Little people: Guidelines for common sense child rearing* (2nd ed.). Shawnee Mission, KS: Overland Press.

Cole, C., & Morrow, W. R. (1976). Refractory parent behaviors in behavior modification training groups. *Psychotherapy: Theory, Research and Practice, 13*, 162–169.

Combs, M. L., & Slaby, D. A. (1977). Social skills training with children. In B. B. Lahey & A. E. Kazdin (Eds.), *Advances in clinical child psychology*, (Vol. 1). New York: Plenum Press.

Conger, J. (1979). *Adolescence: Generation under pressure*. London: Harper & Row.

Conger, J. C., & Keane, S. D. (1981). Social skills intervention in the treatment of isolated or withdrawn children. *Psychological Bulletin, 3*, 478–495.

Cowen, E. L., Pederson, A., Babigian, H., Izzo, L. D., & Trost, N. (1973). Long-term follow-up of early detected vulnerable children. *Journal of Consulting and Clinical Psychology, 41*, 438–446.

Creer, T. L., & Miklich, D. R. (1970). The application of a self-modeling procedure to modify inappropriate behavior: A preliminary report. *Behaviour Research and Therapy, 8*, 91–92.

Creer, T. L., Renne, C. M., & Chai, H. (1982). The application of behavioral techniques to childhood asthma. In D. C. Russo & J. W. Varni (Eds.), *Behavioral pediatrics: Research and practice* (pp. 27–66). New York: Plenum Press.

Curran, J. P., & Monti, P. M. (Eds.). (1982). *Social skills training: A practical handbook for assessment and treatment*. New York: Guilford Press.

Cuvo, A. J., & Riva, M. T. (1980). Generalization and transfer between comprehension and production: A comparison of retarded and nonretarded persons. *Journal of Applied Behavior Analysis, 13*, 315–331.

Danet, B. N. (1968). Self-confrontation in psychotherapy reviewed. *American Journal of Psychotherapy, 22*, 245–257.

Dangel, R. F., & Polster, R. A. (Eds.). (1984). *Parent training: Foundations of research and practice*. New York: Guilford Press.

Davis, R. A. (1979). The impact of self-modeling on problem behaviors in school age children. *Social Psychology Digest, 8*, 128–132.

DeAmicis, L. A., Klorman, R., Hess, D. W., & McAnarney, E. R. (1981). A comparison of pregnant teenagers and nulligravid sexually active adolescents seeking contraception. *Adolescence, 16*, 11–20.

DeRisi, W. J., & Butz, G. (1975). *Writing behavioral contracts: A case simulation practice manual*. Champaign, IL: Research Press.

Dickstein, E. B., & Warren, D. R. (1980). Role-taking deficits in learning disabled children. *Journal of Learning Disabilities, 13*(7), 33–37.

Douglas, V. I. (1980). Treatment and training approaches to hyperactivity: Establishing internal and external control. In C. Whalen & B. Henker (Eds.), *Hyperactive children: The social ecology of identification and treatment*. New York: Academic Press.

Dowrick, P. W. (Director). (1978a). *How to make a self-model film* [Film]. Auckland, NZ: New Zealand Crippled Children Society.

Dowrick, P. W. (1978b). Suggestions for the use of edited video replay in training behavioral skills. *Journal of Practical Approaches to Developmental Handicap, 2*, 21–24.

Dowrick, P. W. (1979). Single dose medication to create a self-model film. *Child Behavior Therapy, 1*, 193–198.

Dowrick, P. W. (1982, November). *Video replay of success versus failure: We don't learn by our mistakes.* Paper presented at 16th Annual Convention of Association for Advancement of Behavior Therapy, Los Angeles.

Dowrick, P. W. (1983a, August). *Accelerating desensitization with self-modeling: Childhood "treatment phobias."* Paper presented at 91st Annual Convention of American Psychological Association, Anaheim, CA.

Dowrick, P. W. (1983b). Self-modelling. In P. W. Dowrick & S. J. Biggs (Eds.), *Using video: Psychological and social applications* (pp. 105–124). Chichester: Wiley.

Dowrick, P. W. (1983c). Video training of alternatives to cross gender behaviors in a 4-year-old boy. *Child & Family Behavior Therapy, 5,* 59–65.

Dowrick, P. W. (1986). *Why behavior therapy is more effective than it is popular: The personality of the psychologist.* Manuscript submitted for publication.

Dowrick, P. W., & Dove, C. (1980). The use of self-modeling to improve the swimming performance of spina bifida children. *Journal of Applied Behavior Analysis, 13,* 51–56.

Dowrick, P. W., & Hood, M. (1978). Transfer of talking behaviors across settings using faked films. In E. L. Glynn & S. S. McNaughton (Eds.), *Proceedings of New Zealand Conference for Research in Applied Behaviour Analysis.* Auckland: Auckland University Press.

Dowrick, P. W., & Hood, M. (1981). A comparison of self-modeling and small cash incentives in a sheltered workshop. *Journal of Applied Psychology, 66,* 394–397.

Dowrick, P. W., McManus, M., Germaine, K. A., & Flarity-White, L. (1985, August). *Using video for personal safety training with the developmentally disabled.* Video presentation at 15th Annual Conference of European Association for Behaviour Therapy, Munich.

Dowrick, P. W., & Raeburn, J. M. (1977). Video-editing and medication to produce a therapeutic self-model. *Journal of Consulting and Clinical Psychology, 45,* 1156–1158.

Dunn, M. E., & Herman, S. H. (1982). Social skills and physical disability. In D. M. Doleys, R. L. Meredith, & A. R. Ciminero (Eds.), *Behavioral medicine: Assessment and treatment strategies* (pp. 117–144). New York: Plenum Press.

Eckerman, C. O., & Stein, M. R. (1982). The toddler's emerging interactive skills. In K. H. Rubin & H. S. Ross (Eds.), *Peer relationships and social skills in childhood* (pp. 41–71). New York: Springer-Verlag.

Ekman, P., Friesen, W. V., & Ellsworth, P. (1972). *Emotion in the human face.* New York: Pergamon Press.

Elder, J. P., Edelstein, B. A., & Narick, M. M. (1979). Adolescent psychiatric patients: Modifying aggressive behavior with social skills training. *Behavior Modification, 3,* 161–178.

Ellis, A., & Grieger, R. (1977). *Handbook of rational-emotive therapy.* New York: Springer-Verlag.

Embry, L. H. (1984). What to do? Matching client characteristics and intervention techniques through a prescriptive taxonomic key. In R. F. Dangel & R. A. Polster (Eds.), *Parent training: Foundations of research and practice* (pp. 443–473.). New York: Guilford Press.

Evers, W. L., & Schwarz, J. C. (1973). Modifying social withdrawal in preschoolers: The effects of filmed modeling and teacher praise. *Journal of Ab-*

normal Child Psychology, 1, 248–256.

Falloon, I. R. H., Boyd, J. L., & McGill, C. W. (1982). Behavioral family therapy for schizophrenia. In J. P. Curran & P. M. Monti (Eds.), *Social skills training: A practical handbook for assessment and treatment* (pp. 117–152). New York: Guilford Press.

Farkas, G. M., Sherick, R. B., Matson, J. L., & Loebig, M. (1981). Social skills training of a blind child through differential reinforcement. *the Behavior Therapist, 4*(2), 24–26.

Feindler, E. L., & Fremouw, W. J. (1983). Stress inoculation training for adolescent anger problems. In D. Meichenbaum & M. E. Jaremko (Eds.), *Stress reduction and prevention* (pp. 451–485). New York: Plenum Press.

Felker, D. W. (1974). *Helping children to like themselves.* Minneapolis: Burgess.

Feshbach, W. D., & Feshbach, S. (1972). Children's aggression. In W. W. Hartup (Ed.), *The young child: Vol. 2. Reviews of research.* Washington, DC: National Association for the Education of Young Children.

Field, T. (1979). Differential behavioral and cardiac responses of 3-month-old infants to a minor and a peer. *Infant Behavior and Development, 2,* 179–184.

Field, T., Woodson, R., Greenberg, R., & Cohen, D. (1982). Discrimination and imitation of facial expressions by neonates. *Science, 218,* 179–181.

Finch, M., & Hops, H. (1983). Remediation of social withdrawal in young children: Considerations for the practitioner. In Social skills training for children and youth, *Child & Youth Services* (Special issue), *5* (complete nos. 3/4).

Finkelhor, D. (1979). *Sexually victimized children.* New York: Free Press.

Frederick, A. B. (1980). How children learn the skill of tension control. In F. J. McGuigan, W. E. Sime, & J. M. Wallace (Eds.), *Stress and tension control* (pp. 231–242). New York: Plenum Press.

Freedman, B. J., Rosenthal, L., Donahoe, C. P. Jr., Schlundt, D. G., & McFall, R. M. (1978). A social-behavioral analysis of skill deficits in delinquent and nondelinquent adolescent boys. *Journal of Consulting and Clinical Psychology, 46,* 1448–1462.

Freud, S. (1963). The analysis of the phobia in a 5-year-old boy. In J. Strachey (Ed. and Trans.), *The standard edition of the complete psychological works of Sigmund Freud* (Vol. 10). London: Hogarth Press. (Original work published 1909.)

Friedman, R. M., Quick, J., Mayo, J., & Palmer, J. (1983). Social skills training within a day treatment program for emotionally disturbed adolescents. *Child and Youth Services, 5,* 139–151.

Fristoe, M., & Lloyd, L. L. (1978). A survey of the use of nonspeech systems with the severely communication impaired. *Mental Retardation, 16,* 99–103.

Frosh, S. (1983). Children and teachers in schools. In S. Spence & G. Shepherd (Eds.), *Developments in social skills training* (pp. 169–193). London: Academic Press.

Furman, W., Rahe, D., & Hartup, W. W. (1979). Rehabilitation of socially withdrawn preschool children through mixed-aged and same-sex socialization. *Child Development, 50,* 915–922.

Galaburda, A. M., LeMay, M., Kemper, T. L., & Geschwind, N. (1978). Right-left asymmetries in the brain. *Science, 199,* 852–856.

Gelles, R. J. (1982). An exchange/social control approach to understanding intrafamily violence. *the Behavior Therapist, 5,* 5–8.

George, R. L., & Cristiani, T. S. (1981). *Theory, methods, and processes of counseling and psychotherapy.* Englewood Cliffs, NJ: Prentice-Hall.

Germaine, K. A., & Dowrick, P. W. (1985, August). *Self-esteem and self-modeling: The impact of (and upon) self-concept during structured video replay training.* Video presentation at 15th Annual Conference of European Association for Behaviour Therapy, Munich.

Goldstein, A. P., Sprafkin, R. P., Gershaw, N. J., & Klein, P. (1980). *Skillstreaming the adolescent: A structured learning approach to teaching prosocial skills.* Champaign, IL: Research Press.

Goodwin, S. E., & Mahoney, M. J. (1975). Modification of aggression through modeling: An experimental probe. *Journal of Behavior Therapy and Experimental Psychiatry, 6,* 200-202.

Graziano, A. M., & Mooney, K. C. (1984). *Children and behavior therapy.* New York: Aldine Books.

Green, K., Beck, S., Forehand, R., & Vosk, B. (1980). Validity of teacher nominations of child behavior problems. *Journal of Abnormal Child Psychology, 8,* 397-404.

Greenwood, C. R., Todd, N. M., Hops, H., & Walker, H. M. (1982). Behavior change targets in the assessment and treatment of socially withdrawn preschool children. *Behavioral Assessment, 4,* 273-297.

Greenwood, C. R., Walker, H. M., & Hops, H. (1977). Issues in social interaction/withdrawal assessment. *Exceptional Children, 43,* 490-499.

Greenwood, C. R., Walker, H. M., Todd, N. M., & Hops, H. (1979). Selecting a cost-effective screening device for the assessment of preschool social withdrawal. *Journal of Applied Behavior Analysis, 12,* 639-652.

Gresham, F. M. (1981). Social skills training with handicapped children: A review. *Review of Educational Research, 51,* 139-176.

Griffiths, R. D. P. (1974). Videotape feedback as a therapeutic technique: Retrospect and prospect. *Behaviour Research and Therapy, 12,* 1-8.

Gross, A. M., Heimann, L., Shapiro, R., & Schultz, R. M. (1983). Children with diabetes. *Behavior Modification, 7,* 151-164.

Gross, A. M., Johnson, W. G., Wildman, H., & Mullett, N. (1982). Coping skills training with insulin-dependent pre-adolescent diabetics. *Child Behavior Therapy, 3,* 141-153.

Gurman, A. S., & Kniskern, D. P. (Eds.). (1981). *Handbook of family therapy.* New York: Brunner/Mazel.

Hall, M. C. (1984). Responsive parenting: A large-scale training program for school districts, hospitals, and mental health centers. In R. F. Dangel & R. A. Polster (Eds.), *Parent training: Foundations of research and practice* (pp. 67-92). New York: Guilford Press.

Hampe, E., Noble, H., Miller, L. C., & Barrett, C. L. (1973). Phobic children one and two years posttreatment. *Journal of Abnormal Psychology, 82,* 446-453.

Hargie, O., Saunders, C., & Dickson, D. (1981). *Social skills in interpersonal communication.* London: Croom Helm.

Harlow, H. (1958). On the meaning of love. *American Psychologist, 13,* 673-685.

Harris, S. L., & Ferrari, M. (1983). Developmental factors in child behavior therapy. *Behavior Therapy, 14,* 54-72.

Hart, B. M., & Risley, T. R. (1975). Incidental teaching of language in the preschool. *Journal of Applied Behavior Analysis, 8,* 411-420.

Hart, B., & Risley, T. R. (1978). Promoting productive language through incidental teaching. *Education and Urban Society, 10,* 407–429.

Hart, B. M., & Risley, T. R. (1982). *How to use incidental teaching for elaborating language.* Lawrence, KS: H & H Enterprises.

Hartup, W. W. (1979). Peer relations and the growth of social competence. In M. W. Kent & J. E. Rolf (Eds.), *The primary prevention of psychopathology: Vol. 3. Promoting social competence and coping in children.* Hanover, NH: University Press of New England.

Hazel, J. S., Schumaker, J. B., Sherman, J. A., & Sheldon-Wildgen, J. (Producers). (1981). *Asset: A social skills program for adolescents.* Champaign, IL: Research Press. [Film or video and manual].

Helsel, W. J., & Matson, J. L. (1984). The assessment of depression in children: The internal structure of the Child Depression Inventory (CDI). *Behaviour Research and Therapy, 22,* 289–298.

Hersen, M. (1979). Modification of skill deficits in psychiatric patients. In A. S. Bellack & M. Hersen (Eds.), *Research and practice in social skills training* (pp. 189–236). New York: Plenum Press.

Hersen, M., Bellack, A. S., & Himmelhoch, J. M. (1980). Treatment of unipolar depression with social skills training. *Behavior Modification, 4,* 547–556.

Hops, H. (1982). Social-skills training for socially withdrawn/isolate children. In P. Karoly & J. J. Steffen (Eds.), *Improving children's competence.* Lexington, MA: D. C. Heath.

Hops, H. (1983). Children's social competence and skill: Current research practices and future directions. *Behavior Therapy, 14,* 3–18.

Hops, H., & Cobb, J. A. (1973). Survival behaviors in the educational setting: Their implications for research and intervention. In L. A. Hamerlynck, L. C. Handy, & E. J. Mash (Eds.), *Behavior change: Methodology, concepts, and practice.* Champaign, IL: Research Press.

Hops, H., & Greenwood, C. R. (1981). Social skills deficits. In E. J. Mash & L. G. Terdal (Eds.), *Behavioral assessment of childhood disorders* (pp. 347–394). New York: Guilford Press.

Hops, H., Walker, H. M., & Greenwood, C. R. (1979). PEERS: A program for remediating social withdrawal in school. In L. A. Hamerlynck (Ed.), *Behavioral systems for the developmentally disabled: I. School and family environments* (pp. 48–86). New York: Brunner/Mazel.

Horan, J. J., & Harrison, R. P. (1981). Drug abuse by children and adolescents: Perspectives on incidence, etiology, assessment, and prevention programming. In B. B. Lahey & A. E. Kazdin (Eds.), *Advances in clinical child psychology* (Vol. 4, pp. 283–330). New York: Plenum Press.

Hosford, R. E. (1980). Self-as-a-model: A cognitive social learning technique. *The Counseling Psychologist, 9,* 45–62.

Hosford, R. E., & Brown, S. D. (1975). Innovations in behavioral approaches to counseling. *Focus on Guidance, 8,* 1–11.

Hosford, R. E., & de Visser, L. (1974). *Behavioral approaches to counseling: An introduction.* Washington, DC: APGA Press.

Hosford, R. E., & Mills, M. (1983). The use of video in social skills training. In P. W. Dowrick, & S. J. Biggs (Eds.), *Using video: Psychological and social applications* (pp. 125–150). Chichester: Wiley.

Hosford, R. E., Moss, C. S., & Morrell, G. (1976). The self-as-a-model technique:

Helping prison inmates change. In J. D. Krumboltz & C. E. Thoresen (Eds.), *Counseling methods*. New York: Holt, Rinehart & Winston.

Hosford, R. E., & Polly, S. J. (1976). *The effect of vicarious self-observation on teaching skills*. (Tech. Rep. Contract No. 8-407674-07427). Santa Barbara, CA: University of California Innovative Teaching Project.

Hull, D. B., & Hull J. H. (1983). Assertiveness and aggression in juvenile offenders. *the Behavior Therapist, 6*(3), 43–44.

Hung, J. H. F., & Rosenthal, T. L. (1981). Therapeutic videotaped playback. In J. L. Fryrear & B. Fleshman (Eds.), *Videotherapy in mental health*. Springfield, IL: Charles C Thomas.

Hupp, S. C., & Mervis, C. B. (1982). Acquisition of basic object categories by severely handicapped children. *Child Development, 53*, 760–767.

Jackson, M. (1983). Adolescent psychiatric outpatients. In S. Spence & G. Shepherd (Eds.), *Developments in social skills training* (pp. 193–217). London: Academic Press.

Jacobson, N. S., & Margolin, G. (1979). *Marital therapy: Strategies based on social learning and behavior exchange principles*. New York: Brunner/Mazel.

Jakibchuk, Z., & Smeriglio, V. L. (1976). The influence of symbolic modeling on the social behavior of preschool children with low levels of social responsiveness. *Child Development, 47*, 838–841.

Jakubowski, P., & Lange, A. J., (1978). *The assertive option*. Champaign, IL: Research Press.

Jakubowski-Spector, P., Pearlman, J., & Coburn, K. (Producers). (1973). *Assertive training for women: Stimulus films* [film]. Washington, DC: American Personnel and Guidance Association.

Johnston, J. M., & Pennypacker, H. S. (1980). *Strategies and tactics of human behavior research*. Hillsdale, NJ: Erlbaum.

Kagan, J. (1966). Reflection-impulsivity: The generality and dynamics of conceptual tempo. *Journal of Abnormal Psychology, 71*, 17–24.

Kagan, N. (1978). Interpersonal process recall: Media in clinical and human interaction supervision. In M. M. Berger (Ed.), *Videotape techniques in psychiatric training and treatment* (2nd ed.). New York: Brunner/Mazel.

Kalat, J. W. (1984). *Biological psychology* (2nd ed.). Belmont, CA: Wadsworth.

Karlan, G. R., & Rusch, F. R. (1982). Correspondence between saying and doing: Some thoughts on defining correspondence and future directions for application. *Journal of Applied Behavior Analysis, 15*, 151–162.

Karoly, P., & Dirks, M. (1977). Developing self-control in preschool children through correspondence training. *Behavior Therapy, 8*, 398–405.

Kazdin, A. E. (1978). *History of behavior modification*. Baltimore: University Park Press.

Kazdin, A. E. (1979). Sociopsychological factors in psychopathology. In A. S. Bellack & M. Hersen (Eds.), *Research and practice in social skills training* (pp. 41–73). New York: Plenum Press.

Kazdin, A. E. (1982). The separate and combined effects of covert and overt rehearsal in developing assertive behavior. *Behaviour Research and Therapy, 20*, 17–25.

Kazdin, A. E., Esveldt-Dawson, K., & Matson, J. L. (1983). The effects of instructional set on social skills performance among psychiatric inpatient skills. *Behavior Therapy, 14*, 413–423.

Kazdin, A. E., & Wilcoxon, L. A. (1976). Systematic desensitization and non-specific treatment effects: A methodological evaluation. *Psychological Bulletin, 83,* 729–758.

Keating, D. P. (1980). Thinking processes in adolescence. In J. Adelson (Ed.), *Handbook of adolescent psychology.* New York: Wiley.

Kehle, T. J., Clark, E., Jenson, W. R., & Wampold, B. E. (1985). *Effectiveness of the self-modeling procedure with behaviorally disturbed elementary school children.* Manuscript submitted for publication.

Kelly, G. A. (1955). *The psychology of personal constructs: Vol. II. Clinical diagnosis and psychotherapy.* New York: Norton.

Kelly, J. A. (1983). *Treating child-abusive families: Intervention based on skills-training principles.* New York: Plenum Press.

Kelly, J. A. (1985). Group social skills training. *the Behavior Therapist, 8,* 93–95, 102.

Kohn, M. (1977). *Social competence, symptoms and underachievement in childhood.* New York: Holt, Rinehart & Winston.

Kolvin, I., & Fundudis, T. (1981). Elective mute children: Psychological development and background factors. *Journal of Child Psychology & Psychiatry, 22,* 219–232.

Kopp, C. B., & Krakow, J. B. (Eds.). (1982). *The child: Development in a social context.* Reading, MA: Addison-Wesley.

Kovitz, K. E. (1976). Comparing group and individual methods for training parents in child management techniques. In E. J. Mash, L. A. Hamerlynck, & L. C. Handy (Eds.), *Behavior modification approaches to parenting.* New York: Brunner/Mazel.

Kratochwill, T. R. (1981). *Selective mutism: Implications for research and treatment.* Hillsdale, NJ: Erlbaum.

Krug, D. A., & Arick, J., & Almond, P. (1980). Behavior checklist for identifying severely handicapped individuals with high levels of autistic behavior. *Journal of Child Psychology and Psychiatry, 21,* 221–229.

Kusche, C. A., Garfield, T. S., & Greenberg, M. T. (1983). The understanding of emotional and social attributions in deaf adolescents. *Journal of Clinical Child Psychology, 12,* 153–160.

Labbe, E. E., & Williamson, D. A. (1984). Behavioral treatment of elective mutism: A review of the literature. *Clinical Psychology Review, 4,* 273–292.

LaGreca, A. M., & Mesibov, G. B. (1979). Social skills intervention with learning disabled children: Selecting skills and implementing training. *Journal of Clinical Child Psychology, 8,* 234–241.

LaGreca, A. M., & Santogrossi, D. A. (1980). Social skills training with elementary school students: A behavioral group approach. *Journal of Consulting and Clinical Psychology, 48,* 220–227.

Lange, A. J., & Jakubowski, P. (1976). *Responsible assertive behavior: Cognitive/behavioral procedures for trainers.* Champaign, IL: Research Press.

Lazarus, A. A. (1977). *In the mind's eye.* New York: Lawson.

Lazarus, A. A. (1981). *The practice of multi-modal therapy.* New York: McGraw Hill.

Lazarus, A. A., Davison, G. C., & Polefka, D. A. (1965). Classical and operant factors in the treatment of a school phobia. *Journal of Abnormal Psychology, 70,* 225–229.

Lewinsohn, P. M. (1974). A behavioral approach to depression. In R. J. Friedman & M. M. Katz (Eds.), *The psychology of depression: Contemporary theory and research.* New York: Wiley.

Liberman, R. P., Neuchterlein, K. H., & Wallace, C. J. (1982). Social skills training and the nature of schizophrenia. In J. P. Curran & P. M. Monti (Eds.), *Social skills training: A practical handbook for assessment and treatment* (pp. 5–56). New York: Guilford Press.

Libet, J. M., & Lewinsohn, P. M. (1973). Concept of social skill with special reference to the behavior of depressed persons. *Journal of Consulting and Clinical Psychology, 40,* 304–312.

Lindsley, O. R. (1956). Operant conditioning methods applied to research in chronic schizophrenia. *Psychiatric Research Reports, 5,* 118–139.

Lorenz, K. (1966). *On aggression.* New York: Harcourt, Brace, & World.

Lovaas, O. I. (1977). *The autistic child: Language development through behavior modification.* New York: Irvington.

Luria, A. (1961). *The role of speech in the regulation of normal and abnormal behavior.* New York: Liveright.

Lutzker, J. R. (1980). Deviant family systems. In B. B. Lahey & A. E. Kazdin (Eds.), *Advances in clinical child psychology* (Vol. 3, pp. 97–148). New York: Plenum Press.

Lutzker, J. R. (1984). Project 12-ways: Treating child abuse and neglect from an ecobehavioral perspective. In R. F. Dangel & R. A. Polster (Eds.), *Parent training: Foundations of research and practice* (pp. 260–297). New York: Guilford Press.

Maile, L., & Dowrick, P. W. (1985, November). *Self-modeling and power lifting: A new approach to peak performance.* Paper presented at 19th Annual Conference of Association for Advancement of Behavior Therapy, Houston.

Marks, I. M. (1982). Toward an empirical clinical science: Behavioral psychotherapy in the 1980s. *Behavior therapy, 13,* 63–81.

Marler, P. (1976). On animal aggression. *American Psychologist, 31,* 239–246.

Matson, J. L. (1982). Independence training vs. modeling procedures for teaching phone conversation skills to the mentally retarded. *Behaviour Research and Therapy, 20,* 505–511.

Matson, J. L., Heinze, A., Helsel, W. J., Kapperman, G., & Rotatori, A. F. (1986). Assessing social behaviors in the visually handicapped: The Matson Evaluation of Social Skills with Youngsters (MESSY). *Journal of Clinical Child Psychology,* in press.

Maxwell, G. M., & Pringle, J. K. (1983). The analysis of video records. In P. W. Dowrick & S. J. Biggs (Eds.), *Using video: Psychological and social applications.* Chichester: Wiley.

McConnell, S. R., Strain, P. S., Kerr, M. M., Stagg, V., Lenker, D. A., & Lambert, D. H. (1984). An empirical definition of elementary school adjustment: Selection of target behaviors for a comprehensive treatment program. *Behavior Modification, 8,* 451–473.

McGee, G. C., Krantz, P. J., & McClannahan, L. E. (1985). The facilitative effects of incidental teaching on preposition use by autistic children. *Journal of Applied Behavior Analysis, 18,* 17–31.

Meichenbaum, D. H. (1977). *Cognitive–behavior modification.* New York: Plenum Press.

Meichenbaum, D. H., & Goodman, J. (1971). Training impulsive children to talk to themselves: A means of developing self-control. *Journal of Abnormal Psychology, 77*, 115–126.

Melamed, B. G., & Johnson, S. B. (1981). Chronic illness: Asthma and juvenile diabetes. In E. J. Mash & L. G. Terdal (Eds.), *Behavioral assessment of childhood disorders* (pp. 529–572). New York: Guilford Press.

Melamed, B. G., Robbins, R. L., & Graves, S. (1982). Preparation for surgery and medical procedures. In D. C. Russo & J. W. Varni (Eds.), *Behavioral pediatrics: Research and practice* (pp. 225–267). New York: Plenum Press.

Michelson, L., Sugai, D. P., Wood, R. P., & Kazdin, A. E. (1983). *Social skills assessment and training with children*. New York: Plenum Press.

Michelson, L., & Wood, R. (1982). Development and psychometric properties of the Children's Assertive Behavior Scale. *Journal of Behavioral Assessment, 4*, 3–14.

Miller, L. C., Barrett, C. L., Hampe, E., & Noble, H. (1972). Factor structure of childhood fears. *Journal of Consulting and Clinical Psychology, 39*, 264–268.

Minuchin, S. (1974). *Families and family therapy*. Cambridge, MA: Harvard University Press.

Mischel, W., & Moore, B. (1980). The role of ideation in voluntary delay for symbolically presented rewards. *Cognitive Therapy and Research, 4*, 211–221.

Monti, P. M., Corriveau, D. P., & Curran, J. P. (1982). Social skills training for psychiatric patients: Treatment and outcome. In J. P. Curran & P. M. Monti (Eds.), *Social skills training: A practical handbook for assessment and treatment* (pp. 185–223). New York: Guilford Press.

Morris, R. J., & Kratochwill, T. J. (1983). *Treating children's fears and phobias*. New York: Pergamon Press.

Morse, C. (1976). The effects of videotaped focus feedback on competency of emotionally disturbed boys. *Dissertation Abstracts International, 37*, 470–471(B).

Mrazek, P. (1983). Sexual abuse of children. In B. B. Lahey & A. E. Kazdin (Eds.), *Advances in clinical child psychology* (Vol. 6). New York: Plenum Press.

Newton-Alrick, G. (1982). *Caring: An approach to sex education*. Salem, OR: DAN Publications.

Nordquist, V. M., & Bradley, B. (1973). Speech acquisition in a nonverbal isolate child. *Journal of Experimental Child Psychology, 15*, 149–160.

Nordyke, N. S., Baer, D. M., Etzel, B. C., & LeBlanc, J. M. (1977). Implications of the stereotyping and modification of sex role. *Journal of Applied Behavior Analysis, 10*, 553–557.

Novaco, R. W. (1975). *Anger control: The development and evaluation of an experimental treatment*. Lexington, MA: D. C. Heath.

O'Connor, R. D. (1969). Modification of social withdrawal through symbolic modeling. *Journal of Applied Behavior Analysis, 2*, 15–22.

O'Connor, R. D. (1972). Relative efficacy of modeling, shaping, and the combined procedures for modification of social withdrawal. *Journal of Abnormal Psychology, 79*, 327–334.

Oden, S. (1980). A child's social isolation: Origins, prevention, intervention. In G. Cartledge & J. F. Milburn (Eds.), *Teaching social skills to children: In-*

novative approaches (pp. 179–202). New York: Pergamon Press.

Oden, S. L., & Asher, S. R. (1977). Coaching children in social skills for friendship-making. *Child Development, 48,* 495–506.

O'Leary, K. D. (1980). Pills or skills for hyperactive children. *Journal of Applied Behavior Analysis, 13,* 191–204.

O'Leary, K. D., & Carr, E. G. (1982). Childhood disorders. In G. T. Wilson & C. M. Franks (Eds.), *Contemporary behavior therapy: Conceptual and empirical foundations.* New York: Guilford Press.

Ollendick, T. H., & Hersen, M. (1979). Social skills training for juvenile delinquents. *Behaviour Research and Therapy, 17,* 547–554.

Panzer, B. M., Wiesner, L. C., & Dickson, W. D. N. (1978). Program for developmentally disabled children. *Social Work, 23,* 406–411.

Parsons, B. V., & Alexander, J. F. (1973). Short-term family intervention: A therapy outcome study. *Journal of Consulting and Clinical Psychology, 41,* 195–201.

Patterson, G. R. (1975). *Families: Applications of social learning to family life.* Champaign, IL: Research Press.

Patterson, G. R. (1976). The aggressive child: Victim and architect of a coercive system. In L. A. Hamerlynck, L. C. Handy, & E. J. Mash (Eds.), *Behavior modification and families: Vol. 1. Theory and research.* New York: Brunner/Mazel.

Patterson, G. R. (1982). *Coercive family process.* Eugene, OR: Castalia.

Peters, R. D., Walters, J. E., & Bradley, E. J. (1981, March). *What's the problem? A component analysis of problem-solving in socially aggressive and non-aggressive boys.* Paper presented at 13th Banff International Conference on Behavioral Science, Banff, Alberta.

Phillips, E. (1978). *The social skills basis of psychopathology: Alternatives to abnormal psychology.* New York: Grune & Stratton.

Piaget, J. (1965). *The child's conception of the world.* Totowa, NJ: Littlefield & Adams.

Porterfield, J. K., Herbert-Jackson, E., & Risley, T. R. (1976). Contingent observation: An effective and acceptable procedure for reducing disruptive behaviors of young children in group settings. *Journal of Applied Behavior Analysis, 9,* 55–64.

Porteus, S. E. (1942). *Qualitative performance in the maze test.* Vineland, NJ: Smith Press.

Poulton, K. T., & Algozzine, B. (1980). Manual communication and mental retardation: A review of research and implications. *American Journal of Mental Deficiency, 85,* 145–152.

Premack, D. (1959). Toward empirical behavioral laws: I. Positive reinforcement. *Psychological Review, 66,* 219–233.

Prince, D., & Dowrick, P. W. (1984, November). *Enhancement of mood with self-modeling: New evidence supporting structured video replay.* Paper presented at 18th Annual Convention of Association for Advancement of Behavior Therapy, Philadelphia.

Putallez, M., & Gottman, J. (1983). Social relationship problems in children: An approach to intervention. In B. B. Lahey & A. E. Kazdin (Eds.), *Advances in clinical child psychology,* (Vol. 6, pp. 1–43). New York: Plenum Press.

Raeburn, J. M. (1985). Towards a sense of community: Comprehensive community projects and community houses. *Journal of Community Psychology*, in press.

Reichle, J., & Keogh, W. J. (1985). Communication intervention: A selective review of what, when, and how to teach. In S. F. Warren & A. K. Rogers-Warren (Eds.), *Teaching functional language: Generalization and maintenance of language skills* (pp. 25–59). Baltimore: University Park Press.

Reid, J. B., & Hendricks, A. F. (1973). A preliminary analysis of the effectiveness of direct home intervention for the treatment of predelinquent boys who steal. In L. A. Hamerlynck, L. C. Handy, & E. J. Mash (Eds.), *Behavior change: Methodology, concepts, and practice* (pp. 209–220). Champaign, IL: Research Press.

Rekers, G. A. (1977). Atypical gender development and psychosocial adjustment. *Journal of Applied Behavior Analysis, 10,* 559–571.

Reynolds, C. R., & Richmond, B. O. (1978). What I Think and Feel: A revised measure of children's manifest anxiety. *Journal of Abnormal Child Psychology, 6,* 271–280.

Rimm, D. C., & Masters, J. C. (1979). *Behavior therapy: Techniques and empirical findings* (2nd ed.). New York: Academic Press.

Rinn, R. C., & Markle, A. (1979). Modification of social skills deficits in children. In A. S. Bellack & M. Hersen (Eds.), *Research and practice in social skills training.* New York: Plenum Press.

Risley, T. R. (1975). Certify procedures not people. In W. S. Wood (Ed.), *Issues in evaluating behavior modification* (pp. 159–181). Champaign, IL: Research Press.

Risley, T. R. (1977). The social context of self-control. In R. B. Stuart (Ed.), *Behavioral self-management* (pp. 71–81). New York: Brunner/Mazel.

Risley, T. R., & Hart, B. (1968). Developing correspondence between nonverbal and verbal behavior of preschool children. *Journal of Applied Behavior Analysis, 1,* 267–281.

Risley, T. R., & Twardosz, S. (1976). The preschool as a setting for behavioral intervention. In H. Leitenberg (Ed.), *Handbook of behavior modification and behavior therapy* (pp. 453–474). Englewood Cliffs, NJ: Prentice-Hall.

Roff, M., & Hasazi, J. E. (1977). Identification of preschool children at risk and some guidelines for primary intervention. In G. W. Albee & J. M. Joffe (Eds.), *Primary prevention of psychopathology: Vol. 1. The issues.* Hanover, NH: University Press of New England.

Roff, M., Sells, S. B., & Golden, M. M. (1972). *Social adjustment and personality development in children.* Minneapolis: University of Minneapolis Press.

Rogers, C. R. (1961). *On becoming a person.* Boston: Houghton Mifflin.

Rogers, D. (1985). *Adolescents and youth* (5th ed.). Englewood Cliffs, NJ: Prentice-Hall.

Rogers-Warren, A., & Baer, D. M. (1976). Correspondence between saying and doing: Teaching children to share and praise. *Journal of Applied Behavior Analysis, 9,* 335–354.

Ross, A. O. (1981). *Child behavior therapy: Principles, procedures and empirical basis.* New York: Wiley.

Ross, H. S., Lollis, S. P., & Elliott, C. (1982). Toddler peer communication. In K. H. Rubin & H. S. Ross (Eds.), *Peer relationships and social skills in children* (pp. 73–98). New York: Springer-Verlag.

Rotter, J. B. (1954). *Social learning and clinical psychology.* Englewood Cliffs, NJ: Prentice-Hall.

Ruben, D. H. (1983). Methodological adaptations in assertiveness training programs designed for the blind. *Psychological Reports, 53,* 1281-1282.

Russo, D. C., & Varni, J. W. (Eds.). (1982). *Behavioral pediatrics: Research and practice.* New York: Plenum Press.

Ryall, M. R., & Dietiker, K. E. (1979). Reliability and clinical validity of the children's fear survey schedule. *Journal of Behavior Therapy and Experimental Psychiatry, 10,* 303-310.

Sanchez, V. C., Lewinsohn, P. M., & Larson, D. W. (1980). Assertion training: Effectiveness in the treatment of depression. *Journal of Clinical Psychology, 36,* 520-525.

Schaefer, H. H., Sobell, M. B., & Mills, K. C. (1971). Some sobering data on the use of self-confrontation with alcoholics. *Behavior Therapy, 2,* 28-39.

Schaeffer, C. E., & O'Connor, K. J. (Eds.). (1983). *Handbook of play therapy.* New York: Wiley.

Schinke, S. P. (1984). Preventing teenage pregnancy. In M. Hersen, R. M. Eisler, & P. M. Miller (Eds.), *Progress in behavior modification* (Vol. 16, pp. 32-64). Orlando, FL: Academic Press.

Seligman, M. E. P. (1971). Phobias and preparedness. *Behavior Therapy, 2,* 307-320.

Senatore, V., Matson, J. L., & Kazdin, A. E. (1982). A comparison of behavioral methods to train social skills to mentally retarded adults. *Behavior Therapy, 13,* 313-324.

Sheldon-Wildgen, J., & Risley, T. R. (1982). Balancing clients' rights: The establishment of human-rights and peer-review committees. In A. S. Bellack, M. Hersen, & A. E. Kazdin (Eds.), *International handbook of behavior modification and therapy* (pp. 263-289). New York: Plenum Press.

Skinner, B. F. (1938). *The behavior of organisms: An experimental analysis.* New York: Appleton.

Skinner, B. F. (1953). *Science and human behavior.* New York: Macmillan.

Skinner, B. F. (1983, August). *Shame of American education.* Invited address at 91st Annual convention of American Psychological Association, Anaheim, CA.

Small, R. W. (1979). Cognitive problem solving and social skills training with preadolescents in residential treatment. *Dissertation Abstracts International, 40* (6-A), 3539.

Smith, L. C., & Fowler, S. A. (1984). Positive peer pressure: The effects of peer monitoring on children's disruptive behavior. *Journal of Applied Behavior Analysis, 17,* 213-227.

Smith, M. A., Schloss, P. J., & Schloss, C. N. (1984). An empirical analysis of a social skills training program used with learning impaired youths. *Journal of Rehabilitation of the Deaf, 18*(2), 7-14.

Smith, R. E., & Sharpe, T. O. (1970). Treatment of a school phobia with implosive therapy. *Journal of Consulting and Clinical Psychology, 35,* 239-243.

Spence, S. (1983). Adolescent offenders in an institutional setting. In S. Spence & G. Shepherd (Eds.), *Developments in social skills training* (pp. 219-246). London: Academic Press.

Spielberger, C. (1973). *Manual for the State-Trait Anxiety Inventory for Chil-*

dren. Palo Alto, CA: Consulting Psychologists Press.

Spivack, G., Platt, J. J., & Shure, M. B. (1976). *The problem solving approach to adjustment*. San Francisco: Jossey-Bass.

Spivack, G., & Shure, M. B. (1974). *Social adjustment of young children: A cognitive approach to solving real-life problems*. San Francisco: Jossey-Bass.

Starke, M. C. (1984, November). *Assertiveness training: Two studies with physically disabled young adults*. Paper presented at 18th Annual Conference of Association for the Advancement of Behavior Therapy, Philadelphia.

Staub, E. (1980). Social and prosocial behavior: Personal and situational influences and their interactions. In E. Staub (Ed.), *Personality: Basic aspects and current research* (pp. 236–294). Englewood Cliffs, NJ: Prentice-Hall.

Stokes, T. F., & Baer, D. M. (1977). An implicit technology of generalization. *Journal of Applied Behavior Analysis, 10*, 349–367.

Stone, L. J., & Church, J. (1984). *Childhood and adolescence: A psychology of the growing person*. New York: Random House.

Strain, P. S. (Ed.). (1981). *The utilization of classroom peers as behavior change agents*. New York: Plenum Press.

Strain, P. S., Kerr, M. M., & Ragland, E. U. (1981). The use of peer social initiations in the treatment of social withdrawal. In P. S. Strain (Ed.), *The utilization of classroom peers as behavior change agents* (pp. 101–128). New York: Plenum Press.

Straus, M. A., Gelles, R. J., & Steinmetz, S. K. (1980). *Behind closed doors: Violence in the American family*. New York: Doubleday/Anchor.

Stuart, C. K., & Stuart, V. W. (1981). Sexual assault: Disabled perspective. *Sexuality and Disability, 4*, 246–253.

Stuart, R. B. (1980). *Helping couples change*. New York: Guilford Press.

Stumphauzer, J. S. (1981). Behavioral approaches to juvenile delinquency: Future perspectives. In L. Michelson, M. Hersen, & S. M. Turner (Eds.), *Future perspectives in behavior therapy* (pp. 65–80). New York: Plenum Press.

Swift, C. R., Seidman, F., & Stein, H. (1967). Adjustment problems in juvenile diabetes. *Psychosomatic Medicine, 29*, 555–571.

Timnick, L. (1982, August). Now you can learn to be likeable, confident, socially successful for only the cost of your present education. *Psychology Today*, 42–49.

Trower, P., Bryant, B., & Argyle, M. (1978). *Social skills and mental health*. London: Methuen.

Uniform Crime Reports for the United States, 1978. (1979). Washington, DC: U.S. Government Printing Office.

Urbain, E. S., & Kendall, P. C. (1980). Review of social-cognitive problem-solving interventions with children. *Psychological Bulletin, 88*, 109–143.

Utz, P. (1980). *Video user's handbook*. Englewood Cliffs, NJ: Prentice-Hall.

Van Hasselt, V. B., Hersen, M., Kazdin, A. E., Simon, J., & Mastantuono, A. K. (1983). Training blind adolescents in social skills. *Journal of Visual Impairment & Blindness, 87*, 199–203.

Van Hasselt, V. B., Hersen, M., Whitehill, M. B., & Bellack, A. S. (1979). Social skill assessment and training for children: An evaluative review. *Behaviour Research and Therapy, 17*, 413–437.

Vaughn, C. E., & Leff, J. P. (1976). The influence of family and social factors on the course of psychiatric illness: A comparison of schizophrenic and depressed neurotic patients. *British Journal of Psychiatry, 129,* 125-137.

Wahler, R. G. (1980). The insular mother: Her problems in parent-child treatment. *Journal of Applied Behavior Analysis, 13,* 207-219.

Wahler, R. G., & Dumas, J. E. (1984). Changing the observational coding styles of insular and noninsular mothers: A step toward maintenance of parent training effects. In R. F. Dangel & R. A. Polster (Eds.), *Parent training: Foundations of research and practice* (pp. 379-416). New York: Guilford Press.

Waksman, S. A. (1984). Assertion training with adolescents. *Adolescence, 19* (73), 123-130.

Walker, C. E., Hedberg, A., Clement, P. W., & Wright, L. (1981). *Clinical procedures for behavior therapy.* Englewood Cliffs, NJ: Prentice Hall.

Walker, H. M. (1970). *The Walker Problem Behavior Identification Checklist: Test and manual.* Los Angeles: Western Psychological Services.

Walker, H. M., & Hops, H. (1973). The use of group and individual reinforcement-contingencies in the modification of social withdrawal. In L. A. Hamerlynck, L. C. Handy, & E. J. Mash (Eds.), *Behavior change: Methodology, concepts, and practice* (pp. 269-307). Champaign, IL: Research Press.

Walker, H. M., McConnell, S., Holmes, D., Todis, B., Walker, J., & Golden, J. (1983). *The Walker social skills curriculum: The ACCEPTS program.* Austin, TX: Pro-Ed.

Wallander, J. L., Curran, J. P., & Myers, P. E. (1983). Social calibration of the SSIT: Evaluating social validity. *Behavior Modification, 7,* 423-445.

Wallbott, H. G. (1983). The instrument. In P. W. Dowrick & S. J. Biggs (Eds.), *Using video: Psychological and social applications* (pp. 73-87). Chichester: Wiley.

Watson, J. B., & Rayner, R. (1920). Conditioned emotional reactions. *Journal of Experimental Psychology, 3,* 1-14.

Webster, R. L. (1980). Establishment of fluent speech in stutterers. In F. J. McGuigan, W. E. Sime, & J. M. Wallace (Eds.), *Stress and tension control.* New York: Plenum.

Weisberg, D. K. (1985). *Children of the night: A study of adolescent prostitution.* Lexington, MA: Lexington Books.

Werry, J. S. (Ed.). (1978). *Pediatric psychopharmacology: The use of behavior modifying drugs in children.* New York: Brunner/Mazel.

West, C., & Zimmerman, D. H. (1982). Conversation analysis. In K. R. Scherer & P. Ekman (Eds.), *Handbook of methods in nonverbal behavior research* (pp. 506-541). Cambridge, England: Cambridge University Press.

Wilson, G. T. (1978). On the much discussed nature of behavior therapy. *Behavior Therapy, 9,* 89-98.

Winkler, R. C. (1977). What types of sex-role behavior should behavior modifiers promote? *Journal of Applied Behavior Analysis, 10,* 549-552.

Wolfe, D. A. (1985). Child-abusive parents: An empirical review and analysis. *Psychological Bulletin, 97,* 462-482.

Wolfe, D. A., Kaufman, K., Aragona, J., & Sandler, J. (1981). *The child management program for child abusive parents.* Winter Park, FL: Anna Press.

Wolpe, J. (1954). Reciprocal inhibition as the main basis of psychotherapeutic effects. *Archives of Neurology and Psychiatry, 72,* 205-226.

Wolpe, J. (1969). *The practice of behavior therapy.* New York: Pergamon Press.

Wolpe, J. (1983). *The practice of behavior therapy.* (3rd ed.). New York:

Pergamon Press.

Yalom, I. D. (1970). *The theory and practice of group psychotherapy*. New York: Basic Books.

Zabel, H. (1978). Recognition of emotions in facial expressions by emotionally disturbed and non-disturbed children. (Dissertation/University of Minnesota) *Dissertation Abstracts International, 38*, 6063(A).

Zentall, S. S. (1977). Environmental stimulation model. *Exceptional Children, 43*, 502–510.

Zimbardo, P. G. (1977). *Shyness: What it is: What to do about it*. Menlo Park: Addison-Wesley.

Author Index

Subject Index

271